Feeding
Your Child

About the Author

MRS. LAMBERT-LAGACÉ, mother of three daughters, sees patients in a private Montreal clinic, is nutrition editor of *Châtelaine*, French edition, and nutrition consultant for *Le Devoir*. She received a B.Sc. (nutrition) from l'Université de Montréal in 1961, is a member of the Canadian Dietetic Association, current Board member of the Society for Nutrition Education, and Chairperson of the Science and Technology Advisory Committee, Canadian Broadcasting Corporation, French network.

Feeding Your Child

From infancy to six years old

LOUISE LAMBERT-LAGACÉ

General Publishing/*Toronto*

Published in 1982 by General Publishing Co. Limited, 30 Lesmill Road, Don Mills, Ontario M3B 2T6

CANADIAN CATALOGUING IN PUBLICATION DATA

Lambert-Lagacé, Louise, 1941 —
   Feeding your child

Translation of: Comment nourrir son enfant.
Bibliography: p.
ISBN 0-7736-1120-7

1. Children — Nutrition.   2. Infants — Nutrition.
3. Cookery.   I. Title.

RJ206.L3513 1982   613.2   C82-094885-3

Published in the United States by Beaufort Books, Inc., New York.

Printed and bound in Canada.

Second printing September, 1983.

Contents

Foreword

NUTRITION IS IMPORTANT at any age but particularly so during periods of rapid growth, during pregnancy, nursing, and infancy. Malnutrition during infancy not only jeopardizes development and health at that age, but may prevent the attainment of full physical and intellectual potential. Conversely, overnutrition at an early age may lead to the multiplication of fat cells, which may make lifelong obesity more likely. This overnutrition, incidentally, is often the result of early and excessively generous introduction of solid food particularly in children who are artificially fed. (Breast-feeding, besides its psychological advantages to the mother and the child, provides the baby with nutrients in optimal proportion.)

Specifically, excessive salt intake in infancy has been linked to hypertension in middle age. Excessive sugar intake throughout life has been linked to an increase in the likelihood of diabetes in genetically susceptible persons. All in all, nutrition in infancy and childhood is or should be a subject of abiding interest to professionals and parents.

Mrs. Lagacé brings to this subject the experience of a well-trained nutritionist and nutrition educator. Known in the field for the clarity of her style, for the care with which she researches the subject and for the sprightliness and charm with which she expresses it, she is particularly well qualified to give the practical advice that is needed. The French edition of her book has been very successful; I trust that this second English edition, fully revised and updated, will be equally popular.

Jean Mayer, Ph.D., D.Sc., A.M. (hon.), S.D. (hon), M.D. (hon.)
President,
Tufts University, Boston

Acknowledgments

LISON CHAUVIN-DÉSOURDY, dietitian, actively participated in the bibliographical research, the study of breast-feeding in Quebec, the review of baby foods, the calculation of the nutritive value of the menus, and the testing of new recipes. For more than eighteen months her enthusiasm and conscientiousness were extremely valuable.

Dr. René Benoit, the pediatrician of my three daughters since their birth, who is associated with Sainte-Justine's Hospital, encouraged me greatly by carefully reviewing the manuscript. His suggestions enabled me to adapt the theoretical to the practical.

Dr. Jacques Letarte, Associate Professor in the Faculty of Medicine at the Université de Montréal, Pediatrician and Chief of Endocrinology and Metabolism at Sainte-Justine's Hospital, also scrupulously reread the text. His comments lend additional credibility to the book, for which I am indeed grateful.

Dr. Jean Mayer, president of Tufts University in Boston, by writing the Foreword, gave the book such a precious seal of approval! I wish to thank him most sincerely.

Dr. Sava Stefanovic, from Cincinnati, provided comments and pertinent information in regards to the adaptation of the text for the U.S. market: his help was most useful.

Cynthia Dougherty, dietitian, doctoral student and mother of a one-year-old, worked scrupulously on the manuscript to incorporate the most recent information for the 1982 edition.

Lise Gauthier once again typed the manuscript with patience, diligence, and accuracy.

To all these valuable collaborators from start to finish, thank you again!

Introduction

AFTER FIVE YEARS on the market and 150,000 copies in print, *Feeding Your Child* had to be revised to incorporate the most recent scientific data.

Rather than inserting changes throughout the entire original book, I decided to start from scratch and write almost a completely new book. This second edition, therefore, contains ten "new" chapters dealing with nutrition during pregnancy, breast-feeding, and a child's first eighteen months of life. The six other chapters from *Feeding Your Child*, which have barely been changed, will eventually form part of a second book on feeding the preschooler.

Since publication of the first edition in 1974, hundreds of parents have asked me questions about various aspects of nutrition for children. These questions subsequently helped me pinpoint parental concerns and better gauge the type of information required. They also contributed significantly to determining the direction this second edition should take.

In addition, during the same period considerable research was conducted to better define the nutritional needs of young children and to evaluate the effects of feeding during the first years of life on the future health of an individual. All these questions have not been answered completely, but several professional bodies and pertinent government departments have developed guidelines on the subject.

This second edition reflects the established consensus on child feeding from conception to eighteen months of age.

It remains a practical and easy guide for planning delicious and nutritious meals, introducing solid foods, and for preparing baby foods at home.

I sincerely hope that the book, in its revised and rejuvenated form, will truly help all parents who are concerned about feeding their children well!

L.L.L.

Feeding Your Child

CHAPTER ONE

The Importance of Feeding Your Child Well

FIFTY YEARS AGO, a child's food was closely scrutinized to ensure normal growth and protect the child from malnutrition. Today, we aim for long-term healthful effects through good nutritious foods provided during the first few years of life. Thus we hope to prevent and even eliminate the two greatest enemies to health: obesity and cardiovascular diseases.

So that readers can better grasp the importance of nutrition during the first years of life, I interviewed Dr. Jacques Letarte, pediatrician and endocrinologist at Sainte-Justine's Hospital in Montreal.

L.L.L.: What are the important considerations concerning feeding and the health of a child during the first months of life?

J.L.: By not giving a child regular cow's milk before six months of age, and by not introducing solid foods until the baby has reached four months of age, the problems of anaemia and dehydration can be greatly reduced.

L.L.L.: Can good nutrition during the first year of life have long-term health benefits for an individual?

J.L.: Teaching the child to choose wholesome foods and to eat reasonable portions is the first step in the right direction. By encouraging good food habits, for example, the risk of obesity is reduced, but this is not absolutely guaranteed. Good food habits should be continued for many years for the child to benefit as much as possible.

L.L.L.: Does a fat baby necessarily become an obese adult?

J.L.: Currently, there are several sides to this question. In 80% of all cases, a fat baby at birth is not fat at one year, and will not necessarily be fat as an adult. However, the rate of weight gain must be watched closely. A baby that gains weight too rapidly during the first year of life has a greater chance of becoming obese over the long term than a fat baby with a normal growth curve in relation to his birth weight.

L.L.L.: Has the theory of rapidly multiplying fat cells during the first year of life been questioned?

J.L.: Most of the research conducted in this area has been done on animals. Very few experiments have been carried out on humans. However, we now know that there are several periods of intense fat-cell multiplication during childhood and adolescence, and that this multiplication is greatest during the first twelve months. If an eight-month-old baby eats much more than he needs, he stimulates the multiplication of fat cells. Although not completely reversible, this occurrence can be partially corrected during the following years when feeding is readjusted to the needs of the child. Irreversible obesity at one year is a myth, whereas normal weight at the end of adolescence is a quasi-prediction of long-term normal weight.

L.L.L.: What are the main points to remember to prevent obesity?

J.L.: The risks should not be abnormally exaggerated, and a fat baby should not be deprived of food or be given skim milk at a few months of age. However, it is recommended that his weight curve be followed closely and the rate of weight gain be watched, especially in families with obesity problems. It is evident that a child born to obese parents has a greater risk of becoming obese than a child whose parents have normal weights.

L.L.L.: Can we prevent cardiovascular problems at a young age?

J.L.: In a family "at risk" (one in which the father, mother, or grandparents have had cardiovascular problems or an extremely high blood-cholesterol level before age fifty), prevention is essential from the earliest years. Cholesterol deposits in tissues start to form in the first year of life, but are reversible up to age twenty. By systematically avoiding certain foods, the formation of "irreversible" plaques can be delayed and perhaps serious cardiovascular problems could even be avoided.

L.L.L.: What foods should be avoided in cases of young children with high cholesterol levels?

J.L.: Egg yolk, organ meats (liver, kidneys, heart), processed meats (pâtés, sausages, salami), cream, butter, coconut, and chocolate should be eliminated from the menu. A relatively strict diet should be adhered to for hyper-cholesterolemic children. In order to balance the diets of such children, their families should consult specialists in the field, and dietitians.

L.L.L.: Can cardiovascular diseases be prevented among children from healthy families by applying the same restrictions?

J.L.: It is indisputable that "moderate" consumption of foods rich in "saturated" fats (meat, processed meats, butter, cheese), and of foods rich in cholesterol, is beneficial for the entire population. On the other hand, there is absolutely no reason to justify significant reduction of eggs, liver, milk, and cheeses in the diets of healthy children. A menu containing less meat, more fish, poultry, fruit, vegetables, and whole-grain cereals, as well as low-fat dairy products, ensures the growth of the child and can limit cardiovascular problems over the long term.

L.L.L.: Tooth decay is a widespread problem among our children. Can it be remedied?

J.L.: This problem can be greatly reduced during childhood and effective long-term prevention can be practiced:
• by avoiding, at all costs, covering the pacifier with honey or syrup to help the baby sleep
• by giving the child a fluoride supplement from the first year of life if municipal water is not fluoridated
• by closely watching the consumption of concentrated sweets by the child, particularly at snack time
• by teaching the child, at an early age, to regularly brush his or her teeth.

* * *

The beneficial effects of sound nutrition don't stop at disease prevention and reduction of tooth decay. One by one we will be featuring in this book the beneficial effects of breast-feeding, the gradual introduction of solids, and healthful menus for your tiny tots!

CHAPTER TWO

Good Eating Habits Begin in the Cradle!

IMPLANTED IN one's memory, eating habits are formed year after year from our taste experiences. Far from being static, they evolve during one's lifetime, always reflecting immediate family influences and the cultural environment. During childhood, these eating habits crystallize around familiar foods and traditional mealtime rituals.

A child who gulps down fried foods and sweets "between commercials" on TV, or who eats few fruits and vegetables and consistently quenches his thirst with soft drinks or colored fruit-flavored beverages, does not retain the same sensory information as the child initiated at a very young age to "healthy" foods.

Developing a taste for food which has undergone a minimum of processing, and which is only slightly sweetened or salted, occurs gradually and painlessly in an environment where varied and healthy eating habits are practiced. On the other hand, it is much harder for an adult to "reverse" previously acquired poor eating habits.

The general attitude regarding food and the various "non-verbal" messages transmitted daily to a child have as much to do with the forming of eating habits as the food itself.

Healthy Foods, Fun Foods

Eating is essentially enjoyable and is as much a pleasure as it is a human need. There are many ways to associate pleasure with healthy foods and, when healthful food habits are repeatedly practiced by the family, the child is encouraged to develop those habits. Therefore:

- By regularly serving green, yellow, and white vegetables, cooked or raw, which can be munched on between meals by everyone, a child will rapidly accept them regardless of the normal reticence typical to the pre-school years.
- Parents' obvious anticipation and expressed pleasure with spring's first asparagus, summer's string beans and carrots, autumn's delicious squash and eggplant, and enthusiasm for a variety of vegetables, will help their children to develop a positive attitude toward these foods and encourage them to try other new food experiences.
- Regular purchases of all kinds of fish and shellfish help familiarize a child with the real taste of seafood and lead him to culinary experiences that go beyond frozen fish sticks or breaded fish cakes.
- Fresh fruit for dessert is readily accepted by a child who has not become accustomed to a regular diet of pies or cakes; to him, fruit is a reflection of the seasons and will never be a "poor dessert substitute for weight-loss diets."
- Frequent consumption of vegetarian dishes based on legumes will subtly dispel the steak myth, while the time is ripe.

To enjoy sound and tasty foods is the best and most positive way to introduce a healthy diet to a child; this obviously implies that parents eat well themselves, but, do not leave out the odd treat. Once or twice will do no harm!

Food — A Source of Physical and Emotional Satisfaction

Fed when hungry, the infant is "physically" satisfied; cuddled and comforted in the arms of his mother, while being breast-fed, he is also "emotionally" satisfied. To any infant, physical and emotional satisfaction is associated with meals and with maternal warmth. Both satisfy two distinct needs — hunger, and the need for affection. This interaction could confuse the child if one is not careful.

The child who is fed whenever he cries, or is overfed to make him sleep longer, cannot, after a few weeks, differentiate between the need to eat and other discomforts. Food becomes the solution to all problems: the need for attention, the need for affection, and the need for diversion.

For several years, Dr. Hilde Bruch, a psychiatrist, has attempted to shed some light on specific eating behaviors (bulimia or uncontrolled eating, obesity, anorexia), and has found that these problems are directly linked to early childhood experiences. When this behavior becomes evident, food does not meet nutritional needs but instead symbolizes almost exclusively the following needs in order of importance or frequency:

- an insatiable desire for inaccessible love
- an expression of rage or hatred
- an ascetic refusal
- a substitute for sexual gratification
- a defence against maturity and responsibilities
- a false sensation of power.

Based upon information collected from many case studies, Dr. Bruch stresses that the hunger mechanism requires proper training to develop normally — we are not necessarily born with large or small appetites:

- we learn to be hungry when it is time
- we learn to know when to stop
- we can easily "unlearn" early in life.

An infant who is forced to finish his bottle or clean his plate is not learning how to control his appetite, while a baby who nurses at the breast for more than thirty minutes is often nursing too long. This means that from the very first weeks a mother can teach a child to recognize various bodily needs and to satisfy them appropriately.

It Takes Two to Recognize Satiety

Mother and child both have a role to play in the normal development of the baby's "hunger mechanism." Although

not a totally dependent human being, a newborn child is capable of expressing his needs and desires within the first few hours of life:
- he can cry, cough, swallow, vomit
- he can smell and hear
- he can distinguish between pain and touch
- he can turn his head in the direction his cheek is touched
- he can twist and kick his feet.

To help the child in his role, the mother must respond to his actions and react correctly to his messages, thereby allowing him to get to know himself better.

A mother who feeds a child to appease all crying, and to console or comfort, is not interpreting her child's messages properly. But, a mother who offers foods in reply to real cries of hunger, contributes to the development of a baby's hunger mechanism. The right reaction at the right moment is one of the key factors influencing the baby's eating behavior.

Should a child refuse to drink the last ounce in his bottle, a mother should not insist he does, but rather respect the child as an individual. When he refuses to eat after having eaten a fair amount, he is saying that he has had enough. This sign of satiety should be respected.

If your baby refuses meat or some vegetable when you start introducing different solids into his diet, you would do better to let him have his own way, and give him the disputed item at another meal, accompanied by some other food of which he is very fond. His acceptance of new foods will only come about gradually, and will need your patience and understanding. To force him to swallow a given food shows a lack of respect for your child. After all, even adults have their little whims.

When there is a loss of appetite, do not force the child to eat because you feel that he must eat to be healthy. Appetites vary during the first years of life. A loss of appetite usually happens when the child's rate of growth has slowed down.

The mother who understands and reacts correctly to messages from her child enables him to participate actively in the feeding process.

Love on the Menu

Ecology plays a vital role in a house plant's development. However, water and light are not the only factors necessary in making it thrive. A plant apparently grows faster and blossoms more readily if spoken to and placed among "good company." Also, certain types of music supposedly stimulate its growth. In short, it is affected by a favorable environment.

For optimum growth and development, a child also has ecological needs which must be satisfied which go beyond the traditional nutritive needs; food alone is not enough. Other important elements, such as parental affection, should be added to the daily menu to create a healthy environment.

This socio-affective "food-environment" association has been the subject of considerable research among children of Latin-American countries, research aimed at minimizing the effects of malnutrition. One of the studies involved weight gain and health status comparisons between one group of infants given supplementary foods during the first six months of life, and a control group of babies from the same Guatemalian village who did not receive supplementary food.

The "supplemented infants," who were from larger, poorer, and less educated families, gained less weight and were sick more often during the six-month period than were the nonsupplemented infants. The extra food did not counteract the effects of their disadvantaged environment.

This somewhat extreme example shows the importance of the environment and of other factors, such as attention and affection, necessary for the proper "total nourishment" of a child.

Another study showed a positive relationship between the nutritional state of young children and the verbal communication which existed between mother and child. The greater the exchange of sounds or language between mother and child, the better was the child's nutritional state. You see, it is a question of a favorable environment!

Sharing Meals

Meals are pleasurable social moments for adults. Not only food is shared, but ideas and feelings as well. To a child, however small, taking part in the family meal becomes one of his first social activities. When he starts feeding himself, the meal becomes a privileged moment during which he sees his father and hears his voice.

Eating with the family does not mean that a toddler must always have what others are eating. Rather, it implies social integration and active participation in a family activity.

The late Doctor Jean Trémolières stressed the important aspects of the family meal when he wrote: "Finally, the very simple rites of the family table delineate those two images without which no civilization has hitherto existed, without which, psychoanalysis tells us, it is almost impossible for us to develop our own personal equilibrium: namely, the Mother and the Father. Food takes on a symbolic aspect, in which its intrinsic qualities are combined with the special qualities with which we endow it."

Mealtime — A Time to Relax

Meals should occur in a pleasant atmosphere, and should not be a time for reprimands, quarrels, or violent arguments. A tension-filled atmosphere can curb a preschooler's often fragile appetite. If a child associates mealtime with battle-time, he will never experience the pleasurable aspects of mealtime, essential to forming good food habits.

A child should never be forced to accept certain foods; he could become a little tyrant should parents try to do so. A meal would therefore become a power struggle between the parents forcing the child to eat, and the child, time and time again, refusing certain foods.

Professor A.S. Neill, well-known author of *The Free Children of Summerhill*, describes in his book *Freedom, Not License* the following phenemenon: "With a child, an eating problem embodies a certain element of protest. The child uses his food preferences at the table to proclaim: 'I'm the boss here, so listen to me.' "

Whims

Without eliminating whims completely, it is possible to circumvent them in order to maintain a balanced diet for the child. No food is completely irreplacable.

A wise mother can substitute one food with another of equal nutritive value without detriment to the child. A child who systematically refuses cooked vegetables will often crunch away quite happily at raw vegetables, and a child who refuses milk will perhaps accept yogurt, cheese, ice milk, or a fruit-flavored milk. In the same way that one learns to respect the newborn baby's appetite for his bottle and his first solid foods, so it is equally important to respect the likes and dislikes of the preschooler. This respect does not imply surrender or an acceptance of the child's whim — rather, it implies a fuller understanding on the part of parents who are determined to feed their child properly.

These whims allow a child to display his personality and individuality, and appear in the pre-schooler at a time when his appetite "normally" decreases. If parents react properly to such refusals and to "momentary whims," and if war is not declared at each meal, a child will give in without realizing it. Being overly forceful about this or that food puts more negative emphasis on a particular type of food and can provoke such a reaction in the child that he will dislike the food for life. This is hardly conducive to the formation of good eating habits.

The more myths and taboos a child builds up about various foods, the more quickly will he close the door to a wide variety of foods, and this makes a sound and balanced diet difficult to attain in adulthood.

Actions Speak Louder than Words

Parents must also be aware of the "logical consequences" of their own actions. At the risk of sounding repetitious, proper eating habits are not acquired at a neighbor's or elsewhere, but by observing father and mother eating three times a day, 365 days a year.

A child who can appreciate the joy of eating a variety of foods from the start does not need to know the merits of vitamin C, iron, or other elements essential for growth. After all, do we wish to raise a child dietitian or simply a happy person enjoying tasty and healthy food?

The following anecdote illustrates the advantages of an approach that stressed "healthy, good-tasting foods" as opposed to a nutrition course adapted to the very young: "I really liked eating spinach until my mother told me it was good for me."

Without knowing it, the child will be conditioned to enjoy eating, and this remains the greatest hope of nutritionists at this time.

CHAPTER THREE

The Prenatal Diet

ALTHOUGH THIS CHAPTER cannot cover all aspects of prenatal nutrition, it nevertheless gives broad dietary guidelines which should be put into practice long before the birth of the child.

Unfortunately, the recipe for a bouncing, healthy baby is not simply two cups of love combined with two cups of hope, left to simmer over a nine-month period. Other elements greatly influence the final product, such as the mother's health before conception, and her diet during pregnancy. It must be remembered that life begins at conception and that an important legacy is begun before birth.

Diet Intervention

Even in our medically well-equipped industrialized society, the birth of a healthy child remains a feat. Many mothers succeed brilliantly; some, unfortunately, lose their babies during pregnancy or at birth; and others give birth to babies of below normal weight, who sometimes have physical and mental defects.

In the United States alone, 200,000 babies are born each year with some kind of birth defect; 85,000 weigh less than 4½ pounds (2 kg). The infant mortality rate for the U.S. in 1980 was 16.1 per 1,000 live births. In Canada it was 10.4 per 1,000 live births in 1980. (Source: Statistics Canada)

In order to avoid many of these problems, and to really help expectant mothers, more and more "diet interventions" are being provided. The results of these programs strikingly underline the tremendous importance of good nutrition during pregnancy. Here are a few examples of effective diet intervention:

- For more than thirty years, dietitians at the Montreal Diet Dispensary have helped low-income pregnant women to plan adequate, well-balanced diets. In addition, they provide milk, eggs, and oranges without charge to the neediest of their clients. From 1963 to 1972, among one group of mothers, the number of low birth-weight babies (less than 5½ lb.) was cut in half, and the number of deaths during the first weeks of life was reduced by two-thirds. The "improved" prenatal diet was not the only responsible factor, but it certainly played an important role.
- In the United States, the Special Supplemental Food Program for Women, Infants, and Children (WIC) is aimed at providing supplemental foods to assist participants in obtaining an adequate diet. The WIC Program serves infants, children, pregnant women, breast-feeding women and non-breast-feeding post-partum women. The program serves approximately 2.1 million women, infants, and children of the estimated 9.1 million potentially eligible on the basis of income. Participation in WIC has shown to be associated with an increase in the birth weight of infants born to women in the program.
- During 1977, the Department of Health of the State of Connecticut analyzed, for a certain region, the mortality rate distribution during the first year of life. It was noted that the babies of mothers given prenatal diet supplements and diet counselling had a three-times lower death rate than the babies of mothers not so informed.
- At Harvard University, the number of low birth-weight babies born in 1977 in four regions of the State of Massachusetts was calculated, and it was discovered that there were nearly five times fewer small babies (less than 5½ lb.) born to mothers whose diets had been adjusted during pregnancy, as compared to mothers whose diets had been left to chance.

A Question of Pounds

To our grandmothers, a pregnancy was almost a dream come true because they could eat to their hearts' content. They accepted the more or less permanent weight gain as part of being a mother, and were thoroughly convinced of the necessity of eating a great deal in order to produce a healthy baby. Doctors burdened by complications at delivery often pointed the finger at excessive weight gain, and that caused an abrupt about-face in prenatal eating habits.

Toward the end of the '50s, a pregnant woman's eating habits were cause for remorse which lasted nine months, as she feared both the scale and reprisal from her doctor; a weight gain of only 5 to 8 kg (15 to 18 lb.) was "allowed." This was a period of tiny pregnant women, mini-babies, and a new series of complications.

In 1970, the Committee on Maternal Nutrition, National Research Council of the United States, recommended an overall weight-gain of 12 kg (27 lb.), a happy medium.

This wise and realistic recommendation was the result of much observation and many scientific surveys which demonstrated that a properly nourished pregnant woman gives birth to a normal-weight baby, with optimal chances for survival and normal physical and mental development. We also know that the weight of the baby at birth generally reflects a mother's diet and her weight gain during pregnancy, and that it can also determine the baby's future development and well being.

A below-normal weight gain during pregnancy is associated with the birth of a smaller baby. Thus, the World Health Organization feels that a baby weighing less than 5½ pounds at birth has fewer chances for survival and for good health than a normal-weight baby delivered at term (3.3 to 3.5 kg or 7 to 8 lb.).

Well-Used Pounds

One might imagine, perhaps, that weight gained during pregnancy goes directly to the baby and that any excess stays on the mother's hips. In reality, it is a bit more complex!

One-third of the weight gained during the nine months goes directly to the baby. The other two-thirds is used for "auxiliary services," the enlarged uterus providing the fetus with a made-to-measure lodging, the placenta becoming a mobile canteen, and the amniotic fluid, a water bed. The 33% increase in the mother's blood content, her tissues and breasts, ensures the baby's better feeding before and after birth. Only a few pounds remain as maternal reserves to facilitate the mother's recovery after delivery and to provide sufficient energy during breast-feeding. In round numbers, the weight gained during the nine months of pregnancy is distributed as follows:

fetus	7	lb.	(3.2 kg)
placenta	1.5	lb.	(0.7 kg)
amniotic fluid	2	lb.	(0.9 kg)
uterus	2	lb.	(0.9 kg)
breasts	1	lb.	(0.4 kg)
blood volume	3	lb.	(1.4 kg)
tissue fluids	3	lb.	(1.4 kg)
fat deposits	6	lb.	(2.7 kg)
TOTAL	25.5	lb.	(11.6 kg)

A Regular Weight Gain

A gradual weight gain during the nine months of pregnancy corresponds more favorably to the fetus's and the mother's needs than a large but irregular gain. The total weight gained is less important than the rate of gain, because the latter has to follow a curve which reflects both the baby's and the mother's needs during the entire pregnancy.

Even if the fetus's growth is slow during the first three months, the energy level required from the internal reorganization of the mother's body, previously referred to as "auxiliary services," cannot be underestimated. A 2 to 4-pound (1 to 2 kg) weight gain is recommended during the first trimester.

During the next six months, a gain of about 1 pound (0.4 kg) per week fulfills the fetus's growth requirements. This means a weight gain of about 25 to 30 pounds for the whole pregnancy.

Weight-Loss Diets Strictly Contra-Indicated

Pregnancy is the not the time to try to lose weight. An overweight or obese mother should not try to lose weight at this crucial time, for a menu containing fewer than 1,800 calories would deprive her of vital nutritive elements and would deprive the fetus as well. A pregnant woman who draws on her body fat for energy to compensate for the lack of food, endangers the physical and mental development of her child. It is better to lose weight *before or after* pregnancy if the good of the child and mother is to be kept in mind.

Nutrition Adapted for Two

Medically speaking, an appropriate diet during pregnancy reduces the risks during delivery, permits the growth of a healthy baby, produces good maternal reserves, and prepares the mother for breast-feeding.

These arguments strongly favor a proper diet and should encourage mothers-to-be to eat better. Many are aware of this but unfortunately, not everyone. A Montreal survey of more than 400 pregnant women showed that nearly two-thirds of these women ate more fruit, vegetables, and milk products, and consumed fewer sweets and carbonated beverages during pregnancy. In spite of these positive elements, however, consumption of liver or other organ meats was definitely insufficient while the consumption of bread and cereal and milk products was slightly insufficient. Other surveys reveal the same findings.

An adequate prenatal diet does not involve that great a change when good eating habits are present from the start. The main changes to the daily menu are practically unnoticeable at the beginning and do not disrupt the family's menu. The portions gradually increase in a pregnant woman's menu, but all additions are derived from the basic food groups and are easily found and prepared.

Regarding calories, a supplement of 100-150 calories per day for the first three months is recommended, and 300-350 calories per day during the second and third trimesters. During the first three months, 100-150 calories can be built up easily by adding one of the following to the daily menu:

III-1: *100-150 Calories More per Day*

- 6-8 oz. (180-250 mL) of 2% milk
  or
- 1-1½ oz. (30-45 gm) of hard cheese (Edam, Mozzarella, etc.)
  or
- I scrambled egg
  or
- 1-2 slices of whole-wheat bread with butter or margarine
  or
- 4-6 oz. (120-180 gm) of fruit yogurt

During the second and third trimesters, the 300-350 extra calories are integrated gradually by supplementing the menu with the required dairy products and other important foods.

In terms of protein, a gradual increase in the intake of protein-rich foods is recommended from the start of the pregnancy in order to attain about 80 grams of protein at the beginning of the fourth month of pregnancy. One can obtain 80 grams of protein by eating daily:

III-2: *80 Grams of Protein per Day*

- 4-4½ oz. (120-135 gm) of meat,
  poultry or seafood .... 30 grams
- 1 egg .... 7 grams
- 1 litre (or 1 quart) of milk or its
  equivalent in dairy products* .... 32-35 grams

- 3 to 4 portions of whole-grain cereal
  products (e.g. 1 bowl of cereal, 1 slice
  of bread) .... <u>9-12 grams</u>

  78-84 grams/day

The "vegetarian" pregnant woman, who does not eat meat, poultry, or fish, but who does take milk products and eggs, will consume 80 grams of protein by eating daily:

III-3: *80 Grams of Protein per Day in a Vegetarian Menu*

- 1 cup of cooked legumes (beans, peas,
  lentils) .... 12 grams
- 6 to 7 portions of whole-grain cereal
  products (1 slice of bread, 1 bowl of
  cereal) .... 12 grams
- 3 tablespoons of nuts or seeds ...... 9 grams
- 1 L of milk or its equivalent in dairy
  products* .... 32-35 grams
- 1 egg .... <u>7 grams</u>

  78-84 grams/day

*I cup (250 mL) of milk = 8 oz. (240 gm) of yogurt = 1½ oz. (45 gm) of cheese

In terms of calcium intake, it is recommended that 400-500 mg per day be added to the 700-800 mg already required in the normal woman's daily diet. The prenatal diet would thus include 1,200 mg in total, which would be obtained by eating the following each day:

III-4: *1,200 Mg of Calcium per Day*

- 1 L (or quart) of milk .... 1,189 mg/day
  or
- 1½ oz. (45 gm) of hard cheese
  (Edam, Mozzarella) .... 300 mg/day
  plus
- 8 oz. (240 gm) of yogurt
  (plain or fruit) .... 400 mg/day

plus
- 1 8-oz. (250 mL) glass of milk .... 300 mg/day

plus
- 4 oz. (125 mL) of milk with cereal ...... 150 mg/day

1,150 mg/day

Besides dairy products, a few foods provide 150 to 200 mg of calcium per serving, such as canned salmon, sardines and makerel, providing they are eaten complete with bones.

It is recommended in Canada that iron consumption be increased by 6 mg, which brings the total necessary for a pregnant woman to 20 mg per day. Since little iron is eliminated once absorbed, the weekly consumption of iron-rich foods that are easily absorbed by the body (organ meats, fresh oysters in season) allows the accumulation of a reserve of this precious nutrient for other days of the week.

In the United States, the Recommended Dietary Allowances recommend the use of 30-60 mg of supplemental iron during pregnancy. The rationale is that the increased requirement during pregnancy cannot be met by the iron content of habitual American diets nor by the existing iron stores of many women.

III-5: *20 Mg of Iron per Day*

- 4 oz. (120 gm) of beef .... 4-7.5 mg
- 5 servings of whole-grain cereal
  products .... 10 mg
- 5 servings of fruit and vegetables ... 2.5 mg

16.5-20 mg/day

The vegetarian pregnant woman obtains her daily iron needs by eating:

III-6: *Daily Iron in a Vegetarian Menu*

- 1 cup (250 mL) of cooked legumes .. 5 mg
- 6 to 7 portions of whole-grain cereal
  products .... 12-14 mg
- 5 portions of fruit and vegetables ... 2.5 mg

19.5-21.5 mg/day

While iron found in vegetable-type foods is harder to absorb, the additional quantities contained in a vegetarian diet help compensate for this fact. Eaten with vitamin C-rich fruits and vegetables, iron is absorbed five times better than it would be otherwise.

A pregnant women requires additional amounts of vitamins and minerals. However, if she regularly eats the above-listed foods, rich in calcium, protein, and iron in appropriate quantities, she also absorbs *all the other nutritive elements in adequate amounts*. Finally, and they are always the same, are the foods which supply the growing fetus its most essential needs:

- a litre (1 quart) of milk or its equivalent in dairy products contributes to both protein and calcium needs
- five servings of whole-grain cereal products (6 to 7 in a vegetarian diet) contribute to both protein and iron needs
- a cup of legumes or 4 to 4½ oz. (120-135 gm) of meat contribute to both protein and iron needs
- five servings of fruit or vegetables contribute to both iron and vitamin needs.

The servings suggested for each food group represent the *minimum* quantities which will satisfy the nutritive needs of a woman well-nourished prior to pregnancy. Quantities recommended in other recent publications I have seen represent maximum servings: these no doubt enable women who are malnourished at the beginning of pregnancy to overcome nutritional deficiencies.

The following typical menu provides a method of co-ordinating all these important foods during the day:

III-7: *Typical Menu for a Pregnant Woman*

With Meat	Vegetarian
1 citrus fruit or juice (125 mL)	1 citrus fruit or juice (125 mL)
whole-grain cereal	whole-grain cereal
4 oz. (125 mL) of milk	4 oz. (125 mL) of milk
1 whole-grain muffin	2 whole-grain muffins
1 6-oz. (180 mL) glass of milk	1 6-oz. (180 mL) glass of milk

1 egg
1½ oz. (45 gm) cheese
raw or cooked vegetables
whole-grain bread
1 fruit

6 oz. (180 gm) of yogurt *or*
1 6-oz. (180 mL) glass of milk

soup or juice
4 to 4½ oz. (120-135 gm) of meat, poultry, or fish (organ meat once a week)
cooked or raw vegetables
whole-wheat bread
1 fruit

1 8-oz. (250 mL) glass of milk

1 egg
1½ oz. (45 gm) cheese
raw or cooked vegetables
whole-grain bread
1 fruit

6 oz. (180 gm) of yogurt *or*
1 6-oz. (180 mL) glass of milk

soup or juice
serving of legumes (one cup (250 mL) approximately)
cooked or raw vegetables
2 slices of whole-wheat bread
1 fruit

1 8-oz. (250 mL) glass of milk

These typical menus reflect the *minimum* quantities of the four important food groups. The menus represent the needs of a sedentary woman weighing between 110 and 120 lb. (50-55 kg) at the time of conception. A more active or taller and stronger woman should increase the quantities in order to better satisfy her higher caloric requirements.

These foods can vary infinitely within each main category and be changed around throughout the day. In fact, the key to success lies in regular ingestion of calcium, iron, protein, and vitamin-rich foods, that is, foods which contribute towards making a healthy baby and maintaining maternal reserves.

Nausea and Heartburn

The fact that the digestion process is slowed down, hormone production is increased, and maternal reorganization favors the fetus's environment, means that the internal well-being of the pregnant woman can be upset. Nausea and heartburn are problems which affect a good number of mothers-to-be.

Miraculous and permanent solutions are rare. There

exist, however, certain procedures to temporarily neutral-
ize nausea and heartburn:

- eat a few soda biscuits or crackers before getting up in
  the morning
- get up slowly in order to avoid sudden movements which
  could upset the stomach
- drinking should be avoided at mealtime: drink between
  meals only, that is, thirty minutes after eating solids
- eat five or six small meals per day instead of three big
  ones and don't go more than two and-a-half to three
  hours without eating a "sustaining" snack
- avoid fried food, coffee, and alcohol.

In most cases, these problems disappear before starting
the second half of the pregnancy.

Are Supplements Needed?

Although a pregnant woman does not require "in principle" vitamin or mineral supplements, many are generally
prescribed. In the "Quebec Nutrition Policy," it is recommended that all pregnant women consume a supplement of
iron and folic acid to compensate for possible poor eating
habits. This advice concurs with other recommendations
published in Canada and the U.S.

In the aforementioned Montreal study on the dietary
habits of pregnant women, the generalized prescription of
large iron and vitamin C supplements is deplored. However, it is recognized that a certain number of women with
deficient diets should be given supplements. Vitamin D and
calcium supplements are particularly important when
consumption of milk and dairy products is low.

Ideally, a medical team should be able to evaluate a
pregnant woman's prenatal diet before prescribing a
supplement; in practice, the attending physician has the
last word.

Salt — Allowed or Banned?

Salt, the long-time enemy of the pregnant woman, is more
often thought of as being something to eliminate rather

than being a nutritious addition to a menu. A number of studies show, however, that the pregnant woman loses great quantities of salt or sodium and that her needs are slightly increased during pregnancy.

A large decrease in salt consumption brings about a defense mechanism which causes tissues to retain water, an opposite effect to what was anticipated.

Alcohol — A Risky Luxury

Alcohol should not be used during pregnancy, since it can cause irreparable harm to the fetus. According to experts, during the very first months of pregnancy consumption of 2 to 4 oz. (60 to 120 cc) of alcohol such as gin or whisky, can affect growth and cause physical and mental deficiencies in one out of ten fetuses. When the amount is increased beyond four ounces a day, the risks to the fetus increase proportionately and dangerously.

If we take into account the serious consequences and the difficulty in measuring the daily dose which would not present any risks, it seems foolish, at the present time, to recommend even moderate daily consumption.

Saccharin: Beware!

As it has been shown that saccharin is a cancer-causing agent in animals, we presume it is equally so when it comes to man. For this reason, a committee of Canadian experts appointed by the Minister of National Health and Welfare in the spring of 1977 strongly advised pregnant and nursing women against the use of saccharin in any form.

In Canada, the gradual banning of saccharin between October 1977 and December 1979 from soft drinks, diet foods, medication, toothpaste, and beauty products, now leaves little room for consumers to purchase this product. Saccharin is only available at the drug counter as a sugar substitute and should be avoided by both the pregnant and nursing woman.

In the U.S., saccharin as a sweetening agent is regulated by the Food and Drugs Administration (FDA). It is still in use in certain beverages, fruit juice drinks, as a sugar substitute, in chewable vitamin tablets, and in chewing gum. Recently, the National Academy of Science's Committee on Diet, Nutrition and Cancer concluded that studies on saccharin do not provide a clear indication of an association between the use of this sweetener and cancer, but noted that several studies "suggested a possible effect in certain subgroups."

Meanwhile, the FDA is awaiting results from ongoing Canadian studies, after which it will publish an order on the safety of saccharin.

Aspartame

Aspartame (Nutra Sweet-Searle, Equal), a protein-based substance about 180 times as sweet as sugar, is available in the U.S. as a sweetener in breakfast cereals, powdered beverages, gelatins, puddings, fillings, whipped toppings, and chewing gums.

In Canada, it is available in low-calorie soft drinks for the moment.

Long-term studies of the effects of Aspartame in people are not yet available: it would seem wise for pregnant and nursing women to remain prudent in their use of this sweetener, in any form.

Other Disputed Habits

From a study that included more than 190 pregnant women, Belgian researchers recently concluded that the consumption of large amounts of coffee (more than 8 cups per day) was associated with a higher rate of miscarriages and premature births. It is, therefore, recommended that coffee and caffeine-rich foods (Coca-Cola, tea, cocoa) should be avoided or at least taken in moderate quantities.

Decaffeinated coffee has also been reported to induce post-natal behavior abnormalities in the offspring of rats.

Certainly further investigation is warranted in humans but it seems wise to recommend that decaffeinated coffee be at least taken in moderation during pregnancy.

When more than twenty cigarettes are smoked daily, a baby's birth weight is lower than that of a baby of non-smoking mother.

Prudence is the Password

The above precautions merely stress the fragility and vulnerability of the fetus with regard to maternal extravagances.

The placenta, the fetus's "mobile canteen," does not have a system which will remove suspicious substances; its membrane is as vulnerable to toxic substances as to essential elements. Properly supplied, it provides an excellent diet. Poorly supplied, the fetus's diet is impoverished, and the development of the child is affected.

A well-informed mother is worth her weight in gold! To obtain additional information on nutrition during pregnancy, I recommend *Pickles and Ice Cream* by Mary Abbott Hess, R.D., and Anne Elise Hunt, McGraw-Hill Book Co., 1982.

CHAPTER FOUR

A Super Baby Food

HUMAN MILK is without a doubt the best baby food, marvelously suited to the needs of a newborn child. Unique since the beginning of time, it is recommended for all babies. Unfortunately, a few generations of parents have erased the tradition, the custom, and its purpose.

For the past ten years, numerous studies on human milk and the milks of other mammals have been conducted throughout the world, helping us rediscover this truly amazing food we temporarily neglected.

A Ready-Made Food for the Species

It is absolutely fascinating to compare the principle ingredients that make up the milk of various mammals, enabling us to fully appreciate how nicely nature makes things.

The protein content in different milks varies according to the normal growth rate of each species. The more protein in the milk, the faster the species grows. The horse, for example, drinks 2% protein milk, and doubles its birth weight in sixty days, while the rabbit, fed milk six times as rich in protein (10% to 13%), doubles its weight in six days! Cow's milk, which contains 3.4% protein, enables the calf to double its weight in fifty days, while human milk, which contains 1% protein, enables a baby to double its weight in more than 100 days, that is, during the fourth or fifth month.

The amount of "protein and minerals" contained in milk

influences the number of feedings necessary during a twenty-four-hour period. The more concentrated the milk, the longer the interval between feedings: rabbit's milk, which is very concentrated, entails one feeding per day, while human milk, being less concentrated, necessitates several feedings per day. Mice, which produce one of the most dilute milks, spend 80% of their day and night feeding their young!

The fat content of the various milks is related to the size of the animal and to the environmental temperature of the natural habitat of the animal concerned. The bigger the animal and the colder its environment, the higher the fat content of the milk. Thus elephant's milk contains 20% fat, seal's milk 43%, and that of the blue whale is 50% fat.

The "sugar" content of the milk varies according to the rate of brain development after birth. Accordingly, human milk contains more sugar or lactose than the milk of any other mammal.

Nature Thinks of Everything

The kangaroo, which carries two young of different ages at the same time in its pouch, produces two kinds of milk: the younger animal drinks a concentrated milk, and when the older one nurses, it drinks from another nipple and receives a diluted milk more suitable to his needs!

The hokkaido monkey gives birth in the spring, and nurses its young all summer. In the autumn, the mother lets the baby forage for himself, and replenishes herself. When snow appears and food is scarce, the young monkey resumes his intake of mother's milk, a seasonal pause.

Advantages for the Baby

Having been comfortably lodged in his mother's womb where he was kept warm and fed until delivery, life is not as easy for an infant after birth. He has to take charge of several functions himself: breathing, maintaining a proper body temperature, feeding himself and then digesting the food, fighting off infections, and so on. These first months of transition between his life as a fetus and his life "outside" call for a proper diet given in an atmosphere of love and warmth.

Human milk fulfills the baby's needs completely. It supplies a baby's nutritive needs, provides incomparable immunological protection, and transmits numerous messages of love and affection.

A. A Marvelously Adapted Food

If human milk is broken down into its main nutritive components and if compared to other milks, it becomes immediately apparent how superior human milk is for children:

- The proteins contained in human milk are much easier to digest than proteins contained in cow's milk or in milk formulas. Once in the stomach, they coagulate into easily-digested tiny particles that are well utilized by the baby, unlike the harder and bigger particles found in cow's milk. Expressly intended for humans and subsequently present in the proper proportion, these proteins are without a doubt better suited to the needs of the newborn.

- The fatty substances in human milk represent not only an important source of calories and satiety value to the baby, but greatly contribute to brain development. Protein usually has been associated with this development, but today, fatty acids are recognized as being equally important; 60% of the solid matter found in the brain is composed of these transformed fatty substances. Furthermore, during the first months following birth, 20% of the brain cells keeps on dividing (or multiplying). Human milk, which contains seven or eight times more essential fatty acids than whole cow's milk, provides an essential contribution.

  It should be noted that human milk does not supply these fatty elements continuously. Less abundant at the beginning of the feeding, they become more concentrated in the last few minutes of feeding at the breast.

This unique phenomenon seems to favor appetite control in the breast-fed baby.

- Lactose, the type of sugar which is naturally present in all milk, is more abundant in human milk than in the milk of any other mammal, and for a very good reason! Once it has been partially transformed into galactose, lactose participates in the development of the nervous system and the growth of the brain, and it also favors calcium absorption.

- Iron contained in human milk was previously thought to be insufficient and present only in negligible quantities. We now know that it is very well absorbed by an infant due to the presence of large amounts of lactose and vitamin C, and because of the small amount of phosphorous and protein found in human milk. Furthermore, it has been found that babies who have been breast-fed rarely suffer from anemia compared to babies fed cow's milk or simulated breast-milk formulas. These last observations, supported by the position taken by the Canadian Pediatric Society and by the American Academy of Pediatrics in 1978, confirms the effectiveness of iron in human milk. The amount of iron in human milk, furthermore, is sufficient for a full-term baby, of normal weight, until the age of six months or until solids are introduced.

- Regarding other mineral elements, human milk contains three times less calcium and six times less phosphorous than cow's milk. Too much phosphorous and calcium will tax the infant's renal system. Found in sufficient quantity in mother's milk, these minerals are important to the development and growth of bones and teeth.

- Zinc is present in large quantities in the colostrum-milk secreted during the first days following childbirth. Even if its concentration is reduced thereafter, the baby is better able to utilize the zinc present in human milk than that added to formulas. In fact, at the present time, it still has not been determined exactly how much zinc should be added to commercial formulas in order to achieve the same physiological effectiveness as the zinc in human milk.

- Human milk contains three times less sodium and potassium than cow's milk which is better suited to the baby's needs and his still underdeveloped renal system. Milk formulas adapted for babies contain equivalent quantities to those found in human milk.
- Vitamin D is present in small quantities in breast milk and was recently found to be "biologically inactive"; in other words, it cannot prevent the development of rickets among totally breast-fed infants, especially if the mother has not taken enriched milk or vitamin-D supplements during pregnancy.
- The vitamin C contained in human milk varies slightly depending on the mother's diet, but it is also manufactured internally by the mammary glands. It supplies a baby's needs entirely.
- Vitamin A and the B-complex vitamins are found in sufficient amounts in human milk as well as in cow's milk and formulas.

Human milk has a nutritive quality which never ceases to amaze. A breast-fed baby does not require additional consumption of water, as his water reserves are adequate after drinking human milk. This is even true for hot and humid days. Milk from a mother who has delivered a premature baby contains more proteins than that of a mother whose baby was born at term, thus satisfying the greater protein needs of a premature baby. This milk, however, does not contain sufficient quantities of all the nutrients needed to satisfy the immense requirements of a very small premature baby, but is nevertheless better suited to the needs of a premature infant than any other milk formula.

B. Happy Effects

The numerous nutritive benefits of human milk are reflected by the general state of health of the infant. Any health professional knows this.

In the Eastern Townships region of Quebec, certain effects of breast-feeding on the baby's well-being were verified. A small amount of blood was taken from 556 infants; some were breast-fed, some bottle-fed. It was found that at six months and at one year the breast-fed babies' blood contained greater quantities of folic acid and vitamins A, E, and C than that of the other babies. Another study made of babies under six months of age revealed that the breast-fed babies had a better weight for their age and were better developed than bottle-fed babies.

In Cooperstown, New York, the medical records of 503 infants who were seen regularly in the pediatric clinic during their first year of life were examined. The advantages of breast-feeding over artificial feeding in reducing illness (otitis media, lower respiratory illness, diarrhea, vomiting) were shown to operate independently of the effect of factors associated with illness such as socio-economic status, family size, day-care exposure, and birth-weight.

The beneficial effects of breast milk cannot be measured — they are innumerable.

IV-1: *Nutritional Data Concerning Breast Milk*

Nutritive elements	Specific effects
Protein	• in less quantities than cow's milk • different quality, better adapted for the baby • more easily digested
Fat	• 7 to 8 times more essential fatty acids than cow's milk • maximizes brain development • more concentrated during the final minutes of feeding, which helps control a baby's appetite
Lactose or Sugar	• in greater quantities than in cow's milk • helps in brain development • fulfills a beneficial antidiuretic role to the mother • fosters, along with the bifidus factor, the growth of as intestinal flora which is resistant to infection

Iron	• absorbed five times better than from a milk formula
	• found in sufficient quantities in human milk
	• fights bacteria as well
Calcium and Phosphorous	• contains less than cow's milk
	• sufficient amounts
	• easily absorbed by the baby
Sodium and Potassium	• contains three times less than cow's milk
	• better suited to baby's needs and kidneys
Zinc	• present in the colostrum in great amounts
	• quantity well absorbed in breast-milk
Vitamin D	• present in small quantities and biologically inactive
Vitamin C	• present in sufficient quantities
Vitamins A and B	• present in sufficient quantities
Vitamin E	• contains four times as much as cow's milk
	• is in good proportion with essential fatty acids.

C. Protection Against Infections and Allergies

It has long been noticed, in industrialized as well as in Third World countries, that breast-fed babies are less vulnerable to all kinds of infections than bottle-fed babies. We now understand how breast-fed babies acquire such resistance.

An infant is born with an incomplete immunological system. He is practically defenseless against his new, hostile environment. At this time, breast-milk supplies a vast arsenal of protective agents which are transmitted primarily during the first days following birth through the colostrum. Each of the substances secreted in the colostrum and in human milk plays a precise self-defense role.

The Immunoglobulins Three immunoglobulins (or antibodies) are present in breast-milk. Two are definitely more active and are manufactured principally by the mammary glands themselves to satisfy the needs of the infant. Unaffected by the action of digestive substances or the stomach's acidity, they line the intestine with an antiseptic material and help the baby fight against pathogenic bacteria, including the polio virus.

The Bifidus Factor A protective agent present in forty times greater amounts in the colostrum secreted in the few days after birth than in milk secreted a few weeks later, the bifidus factor permits the formation of an intestinal flora which resists infection and, by the same action, limits the multiplication of undesirable bacteria. The intestinal flora of the breast-fed baby is very different from that of the bottle-fed baby. Intestinal infections are practially nonexistent in the first group.

Many other substances in breast milk help to complete the baby's defense system.

Anti-Allergenic Properties Rates of infantile allergies are higher in countries where breast-feeding rates are low, and lower in populations where babies are breast-fed.

In the United States, many years ago, a study revealed that eczema, as well as other allergies, occurred seven times more frequently in bottle-fed babies than in breast-fed babies.

The phenomenon is explained by the weak resistance of the baby's intestinal wall when confronted with protein not specific to the species. Breast-milk, on the other hand, supplies only specific human proteins and does not provoke an allergic reaction. Some doctors have succeeded in reducing the problems of allergies in infants from 40% to 7% by giving breast-milk exclusively during the first six months, and by removing dogs, cats, and dust from the immediate environment. This is why breast-milk is universally recognized as the best way of preventing allergies during infancy, especially in families whose histories reveal allergy problems.

Note: It can happen that a baby, breast-fed exclusively, will develop colic as well as skin eruptions. In the first instance, it seems that proteins found in *cow's milk consumed by the mother* are partially transmitted to the baby via the breast-milk, and when the mother adopts a diet which does not include cow's milk or beef, the baby stops having colic. In this particular instance, it is recommended that the mother drink a soya-based formula (Isomil, Prosobee) to eliminate the problem until the baby is able to tolerate the protein contained in cow's milk, at about six months of age. A dietetic consultation will provide appropriate readjustment of the maternal diet.

In the second instance, a baby of a few months of age, who suddenly develops dermatitis (severe skin irritation), might not be receiving enough zinc through breast-feeding, since the amount of zinc found in breast-milk can vary enormously from one mother to another. This can be corrected by adding foods rich in zinc to the maternal diet such as oysters (fresh, frozen, or canned), liver or wheat germ, and by applying a zinc-based ointment to the baby's skin.

D. A Source of Exceptional Contact

Breast-milk is not only a food which is marvelously well suited to the needs of the baby, as well as providing an anti-infection and anti-allergenic defense system, but it also permits the blossoming of a unique relationship between mother and child.

For several years now, the medical field has not only been trying to save lives and to assure average physical growth, but also has been looking at ways to foster favorable global development of the child. Subsequently several doctors, such as Marshall Klaus and John Kennel, have been looking into the origin of the interaction between the newborn and his parents.

Struck by the high incidence of abandoned or abused children, and by the slow growth of children separated from their parents during the first months of life, these doctors have tried to discover a common element for these situations. During their research, they found a common denominator between the absence of physical contact between mother and child during the first days of life and a higher frequency of a number of problems.

The less often a mother took her child in her arms, the less eye contact and the less warmth there was between the two of them. Subsequently, more developmental and health problems occurred in the child.

The minutes and days following birth are key times to initiate and seal the mother-child relationship. Breast-feeding immediately after delivery, or within a few hours, permits establishment of this physical contact. The whole breast-feeding period reinforces this unique relationship.

It is undoubtedly possible to establish a happy mother-child relationship without breast-feeding one's child, but isn't breast-feeding the ideal way to do so?

Advantages for the Mother

The baby is without a doubt the winner when it comes to breast-feeding, which is absolutely normal. However, the mother reaps some dividends as well. Before drawing up a list I would like to tell you about Mrs. Thomas, a nurse in her sixties from Iowa City, who is Doctor Fomon's assistant. Mrs. Thomas, who works with young mothers in her region, constantly tells her charges that breast-milk is perfect. Says Mrs. Thomas:

"It is always at the proper temperature;
It is easily transported to a picnic;
It does not attract cats;
It comes in attractive containers!"

Mothers should truly realize the real benefits to themselves of breast-feeding.

A. A Source of Gratifying Exchanges

We have long minimized or simply ignored a newborn's reactions during the first days and months of life. Recent studies have revealed the mystery of the first hours of life, and the great awakening involved during the first hour following birth. The newborn baby follows human eye contact and reacts to the human voice; he is "ready" to nurse. Far from being passive, he interacts with his mother and participates in the blooming of a privileged relationship.

Nursing shortly after the birth of her child, at a time when the sucking reflex of the baby is at its maximum, helps the mother's uterus to contract, decreases the risks of hemorrhaging, and stimulates the production and secretion of milk. This early feeding seems to be associated with a longer and happier nursing period as well. According to studies conducted with new mothers in Sweden, the United States, and Brazil, physical contact between mother and child immediately after birth promoted a longer nursing period than when there was no early contact.

Breast-feeding is not the only method of establishing this unique relationship, but it is such a natural process that it encourages faster adjustment between the child's and the mother's rhythms — a better synchronization between two beings!

B. Saving Time and Money

Breast-feeding simplifies a new mother's life, saves her money, and makes her daily routine all that more pleasurable! No need to buy milk formula, prepare bottles, care for rubber nipples, wash containers, and so on. It implies a healthy and generous diet for the mother (see Chapter Six), but the price of the supplementary food required during the lactation period is much less than the cost of buying formula.

IV-2: Daily Costs of Various Milk Preparations for Baby

Comparing the costs (in Canadian dollars) of 852 mL (30 oz.) of milk per day

	Price: Fall 1982
A. Breast-feeding (moderately priced diet, extra foods involved)	$0.77
B. Powdered formula (454 g) (Enfalac, Similac, SMA)	$1.11
C. Powdered formula (454 g) with iron (Similac)	$1.14
D. Concentrated liquid formula (425 mL) with/without iron (Similac, Enfalac, SMA)	$1.23
E. Liquid formula, ready-to-use, with/without iron (Enfalac, SMA) 945 mL	$1.93
F. Liquid formula ready-to-use, with/without iron (Similac, Enfalac, SMA) 425 mL	$2.30
G. Liquid formula, ready-to-use, with/without iron (Similac, Enfalac, SMA) 235 mL	$2.51

C. Faster Weight Loss After Pregnancy

About 2 kg (4.5 lb.) of the weight gained during pregnancy is considered to be part of the maternal energy reserves required for breast-feeding. This additional weight is important since it is used in the production of maternal milk and thereby spares the mother's own vital reserves. It is, therefore, used during the nursing period and lost more rapidly when the mother breast-feeds. As a matter of fact, one study showed that at the end of three months a group of mothers who had breast-fed had lost an average of 1 kg (2.2 lb.) more than other mothers who had not breast-fed.

The Trend Towards Breast-Feeding

A survey involving obstetricians and 1,000 mothers in 1976, who gave birth during the twenty-four previous months, was conducted throughout France. This survey clearly indicated an increase in breast-feeding in France between 1972 and 1976; 48% of mothers in 1976 breast-fed their child during their hospital stay.

In the United States and elsewhere . . .

In 1966, 18% of American women breast-fed their baby when they left the hospital, while 50% did so in 1980. In England, the breast-feeding rate on leaving hospital was around 51%, also showing a recent increase.

These figures support the trend in the last decade to a return to breast-feeding in many industrialized countries. The trend is here to stay; note the phenomenal growth of La Leche League International.

CHAPTER FIVE

The Art of Breast-feeding

EVEN THOUGH breast-feeding is an ultranatural act, nursing is an art which is learned and has been traditionally transmitted from generation to generation. Since tradition was broken at the beginning of this century, two or three generations back, training is now done through a doctor, paramedical services, prenatal courses, or through the assistance of La Leche League International.

Breast-feeding essentially depends upon the instinctive reflex of the newborn associated with the maternal instinct, but this process has to be encouraged. In fact, more than 95% of women can breast-feed if they so desire. Unfortunately, certain myths often dispel this initial impetus and turn many parents away from this potentially enriching adventure. It is thus better to explain away these myths before continuing our discussion on the art of breast-feeding.

Answers to these Age-Old Myths

Breast-feeding does not alter the shape of the breasts

During pregnancy, the breasts increase in size and can change in shape long before the nursing period begins if a good supporting bra is not worn, or if the weight gained during pregnancy goes beyond the reasonable limit of 11 to 14 kg (25-30 lb). During the nursing period it is recommended that a proper brassiere be worn twenty-four hours a day, at least during the first few months, so that problems will not occur.

Breast-feeding does not promote weight gain

Certain studies have shown that nursing mothers lose one kilogram (2.2 lb.) more during the first three months following delivery than non-nursing mothers. Understandably, mothers who eat badly and too much, gain weight. Exercise also plays an important role in weight maintenance. If a nursing mother's physical activity is decreased considerably, her weight will vary in consequence.

Breast-feeding is not exhausting

It is a fact that during the first few days following delivery, the baby requires many feedings and much attention from the mother. However, as early as the second week, an improved feeding and sleeping rhythm is acquired by the baby.

In today's society where domestic help is not too common, the young mother has to temporarily forget about dust, fancy meals, and even telephone calls if she wants to keep up her physical and emotional strength! If she eats properly, reduces her usual activities during the first weeks, and if she takes naps whenever she feels the need, she'll readily adapt to the requirements of breast-feeding.

Breast-feeding allows the mother some freedom

Whatever the type of milk chosen, the infant requires a lot of attention and care during the first weeks of life. On the other hand, when milk production is regular and stabilized, toward the fourth or fifth week, the baby can take on occasion one bottle of formula or breast milk kept in the refrigerator or in the freezer (see page 49). When the father or a friend cares for the baby this bottle allows mother several hours of freedom each day, should she want it!

A baby fed breast-milk in a bottle during the first weeks gets used to drinking from a bottle and this helps in the transition period in later months.

The size of the breast — an inaccurate measure

There is no relationship between the initial breast size and the quantity of milk which will be produced and secreted by the mother. In reality, bigger breasts possess more fat, but not a larger milk reserve.

During pregnancy, the mammary gland network of each breast increases due to hormonal changes, and these "little local milk manufacturers" are then responsible for milk production in both small and large breasts!

It is the mother's relaxed attitude which seems to influence the quantity of milk secreted rather than breast size.

Breast-milk does not contain too much cholesterol

It is true that breast-milk contains more cholesterol than cow's milk or formula. Feared enemy of the adult who is vulnerable to its effects over forty years of age, cholesterol, on the other hand, plays an important role in the development of the child's brain and nervous system. The newborn needs cholesterol.

At the end of the first year, after adopting the family's eating habits, there did not appear to be any difference in the blood cholesterol level of babies fed modified formulas during the first six months, and that of babies breast-fed over a similar length of time. Furthermore, the effect of a high or low-cholesterol diet on the cholesterol content of breast-milk has been verified. Whatever the mother's diet, cholesterol-rich or cholesterol-poor, breast-milk does not alter and consistently contains the same quantity of cholesterol. Nature knows best!

Breast-milk is not polluted

A few years ago, the information media reported that PCBs — polychlorinated biphenyls — were found in Canadian, American, and European mothers' breast-milk. In the early 1970s, samples of human milk from two cities in California contained PCB levels of 60 ppb (parts per billion) and average levels in human milk in Germany and Sweden were 16 ppb and 100 ppb respectively. The National Minister of Health in Canada has recognized that PCBs are present in breast-milk, but periodic testing undertaken to control the levels of PCBs has revealed that the breast-milk tested contained PCBs in amounts far below the norms judged acceptable and levels are actually decreasing. Confronted by public concern, two committees of experts, one Canadian, the other American, have studied all aspects of the question. Keeping in mind the present available information, these two committees have come to the conclusion that the advantages of breast-feeding greatly surpass the risks involved by a diminishing amount of PCB contamination. Laws in Canada and the U.S. now limit the use and disposal of these chemicals by industry. As a result of such indications that the PCBs posed a realistic threat to human health, Congress decided to mandate an end to the manufacture of PCBs within the United States in October of 1976. It is, however, recommended that nursing mothers avoid eating fish which comes from the St. Lawrence River and surrounding areas, as well as from the Great Lakes, as these fish have high accumulations of PCBs.

Not all mothers can breast-feed

Even if more than 95% of mothers are physically able to breast-feed, a mother who does not "want" to breast-feed should not do so. In actual fact, there are only a very few absolute medical counterindications which can prevent a mother from breast-feeding. In such cases, the treating physician or specialist is the best counsel.

A badly nourished mother can nonetheless breast-feed

The mother's diet does not influence the principal nutrients contained in breast-milk. Only the volume of milk will decrease in extreme cases of malnutrition. In developing countries, where the mother's diet is often far from sufficient, breast-milk supplies adequate quantities of protein, fat, sugar, and immunological substances during the first three months, although the mineral and vitamin content may be low. In spite of these inadequacies, breast-milk from poorly nourished women is able to assure the growth and initial development of millions of children throughout the world.

A decision which should be made together

In our society, the art of breast-feeding can hardly be improvised at the last minute, after the baby is born.

Even if it is impossible to dispute the superiority of breast-milk, the decision made to breast-feed involves a certain amount of reflection. It is a decision that should be made after serious thinking throughout the pregnancy and even before. It is a joint decision made between husband and wife, to be discussed by the family if other children are involved since breast-feeding alters the family routine somewhat during the first months.

The husband's approval and encouragement should not be underestimated as his overall attitude largely contributes to the mother's calm and serenity. A father's tense or contrary attitude can adversely affect the mother's spirits and could decrease milk production.

Once the decision to breast-feed is made, an exemplary doctor encourages the prospective parents, and supplies information necessary to successful breast-feeding.

Before birth, the physical conditioning of the breast is an adjunct or addition to the psychological preparation of the couple.

Conditioning the Breasts before Delivery

To facilitate the first feeding and increase the elasticity of the nipples, it is recommended that the breasts be carefully prepared during the last trimester of pregnancy. Only a few minutes per day are required. It is simply necessary to:

1. Rub the nipples for a few minutes twice a day with a rough bath towel; or
2. Strengthen the nipple by pulling on it with two fingers, the forefinger and the thumb. The nipples will then lengthen easily and will provide better secretion of the milk after birth. (The extending of the nipple can provoke a slight secretion of a yellowish liquid, colostrum, the forerunner of real breast-milk. This secretion is perfectly normal. By washing the nipple as indicated below, there is absolutely no problem.)
3. Wash the nipples daily with warm water: this prevents the irritation and drying of the nipples which can be caused by the secretions.
4. A lanoline-based cream can be applied to the nipples to prevent irritation and dryness.

While at the hospital:
- During delivery, avoid as much as possible the use of sedatives, since their use decreases the baby's reflexes at birth.
- As soon as the baby is born, he/she should be breast-fed, since it is during this first hour of life that the baby's sucking reflex is at its maximum. This early sucking activates the mechanism for the production of breast-milk.
- It is preferable that the baby "live-in" to allow feeding on demand. During the first days which are days of learning and adaptation, the feedings should be numerous, as many as ten the first day. This will stimulate production and secretion of the milk and satisfy the baby's need for warmth and tenderness.
- Find the most comfortable nursing position with the help of a nurse. Nurse no more than five minutes at each

breast during each feeding on the first day. Offer both breasts at each feeding starting with the breast offered last at the preceding feeding.

- Gradually increase the length of each feeding each day.
- Never interrupt the baby while he is actively feeding to burp him — wait until he pauses. This will enable him to reject the bubbles he has swallowed.
- Never give the baby a bottle of formula or sweetened water between feedings. This decreases the baby's appetite and disrupts the still fragile milk production process.
- During the entire lactation period, support the breasts with a good-quality cotton nursing brassiere which opens to adequately expose a large part of the breast, not only the nipple. Avoid use of plastic or rubber-lined brassieres which irritate the nipples because they trap excess moisture.

The Art of Nursing on Demand

Following a number of personal accounts and a conversation with a La Leche League monitor, I became convinced of the importance of nursing on demand, without a fixed timetable. At first, this arrangement seems to require the mother to be available at all times but, as the weeks pass, mother and child comply to a jointly satisfactory rhythm and, when the needs of the newborn are considered during the first days of life, the benefits of such an arrangement are widely appreciated.

During the first hours of life, the child is wide-awake and is "actively" discovering his new environment. He reacts to this environment. His sucking reflex is particularly well developed following the first few minutes of delivery. As mentioned previously, during the first twenty-four hours of life the baby should nurse as many as ten times and perhaps even more. The mother who can respond to the appetite requirements of the baby by having him live-in satisfies her baby while helping herself, since these small but numerous feedings initiate a good milk supply. A number of studies associate part of the success of breast-feeding with the first feeding, given immediately after delivery or within the first hours of the infant's life. Other observations conclude that the baby who is close to his mother from the start finds an acceptable biorythm more rapidly, and his nursing and sleeping schedules are spaced more regularly.

The great awakening of the first hours now over, the baby falls into a deep sleep, and more intense cries are heard only around the third day. This ritual peculiar to the newborn entails that the mother be initially alert and available, but underlines as well the necessity to abandon a fixed nursing schedule at three- or four-hour intervals during this key period.

Gradually the baby is able to take larger and larger quantities of milk at one time, and his digestive system is also better adapted. At the end of a few weeks, he normally acquires a certain regularity and three or four hours can lapse between feedings. He can often sleep six consecutive hours between two feedings, once every twenty-four hours . . . Blessed are parents whose baby chooses the night for this prolonged nap!

As the entire breast-feeding process is an interaction between mother and child, after a few weeks the two adapt to a satisfactory way of living, without a rigid schedule.

One small precautionary message regarding breast-feeding on demand: interpretation of the baby's crying is very important, since crying does not always signal hunger. To feed a baby at the least bit of crying can involve serious long-term consequences!

A compromise between total feeding on demand and the fixed schedule seems to me to be acceptable after the first few weeks in order to respect the physical needs of the child as well as the psychological needs of the mother.

This compromise implies that certain feedings are given at more or less regular intervals during the day (10 o'clock, 1 o'clock, 4 o'clock, and 7 o'clock). The others (the first feeding in the morning and the last feeding of the evening) are given according to the baby's requests. This schedule should be flexible and comprehensive. If the baby is sleeping soundly at 1 o'clock, he can be fed at 1:30, and the following feeding is given at 4:30 P.M. rather than at 4 P.M.

To each her own schedule . . . A happy mother is twice as valuable!

Problem Areas and Solutions

It goes without saying that the return home requires further adaptation on the part of the mother and her infant. Four or five days after delivery, milk production is not yet stabilized, and learning about breast-feeding is still continuing. The nights are short and the days long . . . sometimes there are problems, but they are rarely without a solution.

Breast congestion

Breast congestion, or engorgement, can occur at the beginning of the breast-feeding regimen if the breasts are not completely emptied after each nursing or if the feedings are too far apart. A hot-water compress quickly relieves the engorged breast. A breast which is too full leaves little of the nipple for the baby to suck on. In order to enable him to drink easily, it is suggested that milk be manually expressed before or after nursing.

Cracked, fissured, or split nipples

Nipples can crack, fissure or split, particularly in women with delicate, pale skin, in spite of proper preparation of the breasts during pregnancy. To reduce discomfort, a lanolin-based cream is applied on the nipple and nursing is limited to five to seven minutes per nipple at each feeding for a few days. After each nursing period, the nipple is dried and left exposed to the air for a fifteen-minute period.

Breast infection or mastitis

Breast infection is usually present when the mother complains that she is really exhausted, has painful breasts, and a fever. Rest is the best medicine, as well as frequent breast-feeding which will decongest the breast. Should the fever persist, the doctor can prescribe antibiotics which will not prevent the continuation of breast-feeding.

Insufficient milk

An insufficient supply of milk is without a doubt the greatest source of worry and one of the main causes of the premature abandonment of breast-feeding. This milk shortage, usually short-lived, is ordinarily associated with fatigue, anxiety, or a greater demand by the baby caused by a growth spurt. When one realizes that nursing mothers of twins are well able to provide for their babies, confidence in a mother's ability to nurse one child is quickly regained.

On the other hand, we should realize that if the nursing mother reduces her food consumption, thinking that she will be able to lose weight faster, she can involuntarily decrease her milk supply considerably.

Rest, an adequate diet (see Chapter Six), a refreshing shower or a warm relaxing bath before breast-feeding, accompanied occasionally by a small glass of wine or beer, are but a few ways to restore confidence and relaxation in the temporarily distressed nursing mother.

Another method of increasing milk production is by increasing the number of feedings for a few days which stimulates milk production and better corresponds to the increased appetite needs of the baby.

Freezing Breast-Milk

The freezing of breast-milk has long been carried on by milk-bank organizations responsible for preserving this precious liquid, donated by nursing mothers in various regions in order to supply milk for premature, hospitalized, or ailing babies.

However, the home-freezing of breast-milk is a relatively new development. It is a simple technique and, while it remains one of the most efficient in food preservation, it is one which is widely available to everyone. Thanks to the home-freezing of breast-milk, more freedom is available to the mother and it enables the father to feed his baby without the child having to change his high-quality diet. This also permits the mother of a hospitalized premature baby to provide at a distance for his nutritive and immunological needs.

It is recommended that the milk be manually expressed. Certain hygienic rules should be observed in order to avoid contaminating the breast-milk. Let us proceed by stages:

1. Generously pour boiling water into a pyrex measuring cup or other container to be used for the milk. Leave it for two to three minutes in order to sterilize it, then pour out.

2. Prepare a small polyethylene bag (those used in certain types of baby bottles), and label the date of collection with a self-adherent tag.

3. Before extracting the milk, wash hands and nipples.

4. Gently massage the breast and the nipple in order to stimulate the "let down reflex."

5. Express the milk by placing the thumb and forefinger around the nipple — at first, this may take some time, but with practice, several ounces can be expressed in about fifteen minutes.

6. Pour the milk from the "sterilized" collecting cup into the polyethylene bag.

7. Seal the bag well and refrigerate immediately.

8. Once the bag of milk has cooled, after about an hour in the refrigerator, place it in the rear of the freezer, away from the door, in order to ensure that the temperature is very cold and uniform. In the refrigerator, breast-milk can keep for a maximum of two days; in the freezer, breast-milk may be kept for two to six months.

9. To warm the milk, take out from the freezer and place the bag in a container of warm water for five minutes. Shake the milk to evenly distribute the fat particles and serve at once!

10. Once thawed, but not warmed, breast-milk can be kept in the refrigerator for one day.

Length of Breast-Feeding Period

Health professionals agree that breast-milk suffices by itself in adequately providing for the nutritive needs of the baby for the first four to six months of life, as long as the baby is born at term, is of normal weight, and in good health.

No one limits the breast-feeding period to six months; breast-milk can complement the baby's diet for several years, should the mother desire to do so. We simply emphasize that the maximum contribution of breast-milk as the only item in a baby's diet is during the first four to six months of life.

In reality, the duration of the breast-feeding period, whether two weeks, one month or two, does not matter; the experience is worthwhile for both parties, mother and child. Breast-milk is still the most marvelously well-adapted food for baby and the most readily accessible for the mother. Results of a large mail and telephone survey conducted in the United States in 1980 revealed that 25% of infants are still breast-fed at six months of age, 19% at eight months, 10% at ten months and over 7% at twelve months. Many are the mothers, whose experiences have not been statistically recorded and who have successfully breast-fed for six months, who have taken time to write me of their success!

Thanks to the advantage of freezing a reserve of breast-milk as soon as milk production is adequate to do so, breast-feeding can become compatible with a flexible work schedule after about three months.

Weaning is a sensitive time to go through. Ideally this transition period is a gentle one, slow and gradual, with little upset for both baby and mother.

If the child is six or seven months old, he gradually leaves the breast and adapts to a cup containing whole-milk or formula. If the baby is but a few weeks or months old, he gradually gives up breast-milk for formula. Three weeks should be allowed for the change.

One method is to substitute one bottle-feeding for one breast-feeding every four or five days, keeping the morning and night feeding at the breast. Let go of the morning nursing before the night one. By decreasing the number of breast-feeding periods, milk production is automatically reduced and the mother's adaptation period is facilitated.

Another method involves reducing each feeding by five minutes, that is two and one-half minutes per breast. Feeding is then completed by giving three ounces of formula in a bottle. Five days after the first decrease, the length of the nursing period is again cut by five minutes, and four ounces of formula is offered after nursing. The process is continued until the formula entirely replaces breast-milk.

To obtain additional information about breast-feeding, the following books are available:

1. *The Complete Book of Breastfeeding*
   Marvin S. Eiger, M.D., and Sally Wendkos Olds
   Workman Pub. Co., 1972

2. *The Womanly Art of Breastfeeding*
   La Leche League International, 3rd edition, 1981

3. *Nursing Your Baby*
   Karen Pryor
   Harper and Row, 1975

CHAPTER SIX

The Nursing Mother's Diet

THANKS TO THE efficient work of the mammary glands and the mother's adequate diet, a breast-fed baby receives the ideal food in terms of both quality and quantity.

After thorough examination of the composition of breast-milk in Chapter Four, we can now turn our attention to the diet of the "producer" who is responsible for the production of this "super" baby food. It is important to stress that the mother's diet influences not only the quality, but also the quantity, of milk secreted by the mammary glands. As previously stated, however, breast-milk cannot be *significantly* altered in quality or quantity except in extreme cases of malnutrition. In fact, even in developing countries nursing mothers are able to produce milk which contains sufficient amounts of protein, fat, and lactose (sugar) during the first few months following delivery. When there is severe malnutrition, it is the quantity of the milk which is insufficient, not the essential ingredients.

However, in most situations a nursing mother who eats well produces milk which is richer in vitamins than milk produced by a mother who is malnourished. Moreover, the well-fed mother does not endanger her own reserves, a fact which should not be understated.

This said, the nursing mother's diet is not complicated. It is made up of the same good foods which were found to be so important during pregnancy (Chapter Three), but in slightly larger quantities.

150-200 More Calories

The nutritive needs of the newborn are greater than during his fetal life. The caloric intake in the nursing mother's diet should, therefore, be slightly higher than during her pregnancy if she wants to manufacture sufficient quantities of milk. In relation to the energy demands during pregnancy, an *additional* daily supplement of 150-200 calories is required; this represents an increase of 450-500 calories in the diet of the nursing mother since she became pregnant. This caloric surplus seems like a small amount to supply 16 to 30 ounces (480 to 825 mL) of milk per day, but this is not the only source of calories.

The 4.4 to 6.6 pounds of fat deposits (two to three kilos), or more, deposited in the maternal organism during the gestation period and kept throughout the delivery period, are used at a rate of about 300 calories per day as an additional source of energy. Slowly but surely, these fat deposits disappear, used for the benefit of the baby during the first three or four months.

A daily diet containing between 2,200 to 2,500 calories seems to satisfy both mother's and baby's needs. This can be even more generous depending on the mother's dietary habits and her level of physical activity.

Key Foods Found on the Daily Menu

The suggested portions for each food group represent the *minimum* quantities capable of satisfying the nutritive needs of a well-fed woman before and during pregnancy.

Milk Products

Without a doubt, milk products represent a food group which is particularly essential to mother and child during the nursing period. A litre (1 quart) of milk per day or its equivalent in milk products is the minimum daily amount required to supply all the calcium needed for tooth and bone formation in the baby, while still conserving the mother's own reserves. As a complementary contribution, a litre (1 quart) of milk supplies more than 32-35 grams of complete protein, a good quantity of B vitamins, and the entire daily vitamin D requirement. Be sure to buy a vitamin-D enriched milk if living in the United States; enrichment with this vitamin is not compulsory.

An eight-ounce glass of milk (250 mL) can be replaced by:

1½ oz. (45 gm) of cheese
or
8 oz. (240 gm) of yogurt
or
8 oz. (250 mL) of milk-based soup or dessert
or
2 scoops of ice cream or ice milk (occasionally)

Meat, Poultry, Fish, or Substitute

One daily serving of 4 to 4½ oz. of meat, poultry, or fish is ample in supplying a sufficient quantity of protein, B vitamins and iron.

A weekly meal of liver, kidney, or fresh oysters supplies an additional amount of iron and zinc, useful nutritive elements needed by the nursing mother.

One or more cups of cooked dried vegetables (soya beans, dried peas, lentils, etc.) supplies the vegetarian nursing mother with good quality vegetable protein which becomes even more effective in building and repairing tissues if eaten with whole-grain cereal or bread.

Eggs

Four to seven eggs are recommended for the nursing mother. Two can replace a serving of meat. Eggs contain easily assimilated protein and supply vitamins and minerals. Their contribution should not be underestimated, nor should they be eliminated from the menu because of their high cholesterol content. According to many researchers studying atherosclerosis, it is the total quantity of "saturated" fats which affects the cholesterol level in the blood. Instead of eliminating eggs entirely from the diet, it would be better to watch the portions of meat, cheese, butter or margarine.

Whole-grain Cereal and Bread

The "carnivorous" nursing mother should eat four to six slices of whole-grain bread or its equivalent in cereal products every day. Bread not only rounds off the total number of calories, but supplies a significant quantity of protein, iron, and B vitamins.

The "vegetarian" nursing mother should eat six to eight portions of bread or cereal products every day in order to complete the legume protein and to supply additional iron, B vitamins, and calories.

A slice of whole-grain bread can be replaced by:

one bowl of whole-grain cereal, cooked or ready-to-eat
or
½ cup (125 mL) of brown or parboiled rice
or
½ cup (125 mL) of enriched pastas
or
one whole-wheat or bran muffin
or
one whole-wheat, buckwheat or oatmeal pancake

Fruit

Overflowing with vitamins, minerals, food fiber and "permissible" sugar, fruits play an appealing role in the nursing mother's diet. They supply color and flavor without tilting the scales the wrong way. Two portions per day represent a *minimum* amount.

Whether fresh, frozen, or canned, fruits are a winning part of any meal. Several kinds of fruit are now available, and canned without sugar or canned in unsweetened fruit juice represent valid choices when fresh fruit is too expensive.

Fruits rich in vitamin C, such as oranges, grapefruits, strawberries, and melons, should be eaten every day and are a welcome addition to a vegetarian diet based on cereals or legumes, since they enhance iron absorption.

It is well known that iron is an important nutrient in the proper functioning of the organism. As all precious substances seem to be, however, iron is especially vulnerable particularly in a meatless diet. Since vitamin C can increase the absorption of iron from foods, notably vegetables, consumption of fruit and vegetables at each meal is very beneficial in a vegetarian diet.

Vegetables

A food without fault which contains a great number of nutrients and few calories, yellow, green, red or white, cooked or raw, in juice or in soup form, all vegetables add color and texture to our meals. Whether they are fresh, frozen, or canned, they contribute to the daily nutritional food balance.

Three servings per day represent minimum rations. Additional supplementary portions are always an added health benefit.

Fats

A moderate quantity of butter, margarine that has been only partially hydrogenated, or polyunsaturated oil (corn, sunflower, etc.) complete the menu. Used in moderation for cooking, as a spread or as a dressing, fats add useful calories while aiding in the absorption of several vitamins.

A diet which contains a larger amount of polyunsaturated fats than saturated fats has a parallel influence on breast-milk. Vegetarian nursing mothers who consume neither milk products, meat, or eggs, produce milk which is richer in polyunsaturated fats than "carnivorous" nursing mothers.

A nursing mother need not adopt such an "extreme" diet, however, since human milk naturally contains an appreciable amount of unsaturated fats, as much as five times more than cow's milk.

Breast-milk resists reflecting fluctuations in the intake

of cholesterol in the nursing mother's diet. Whether the diet be high or low in cholesterol, the amount of cholesterol in breast-milk remains relatively stable, responding to nature's requirements and actively working at developing the baby's brain and nervous sytem.

Liquids

Contrary to popular belief, liquids consumed by a mother do not directly influence breast-milk production. As a baby is the first to be "served," it is the mother who runs the risk of suffering from an insufficient amount of liquids and becoming dehydrated.

If milk products are consumed in the form of liquid milk, if one of the day's fruits is taken in juice form, and if soup or vegetable juice is added to the menu, a few glasses of water are all that remain to be taken each day.

However, if foods are eaten mainly in solid form (cheese, stewed fruits, or cooked vegetables), it will then be necessary to drink several glasses of water between and at meals in order to maintain the water reserves essential to the proper functioning of the maternal organism.

Sweets, Pastries, and Others

If one wishes to give priority to the key food elements useful to both the mother and the baby during this crucial period, and if at the same time one wants to avoid consumption of "useless" calories, there then remains little place for sweets, pastries, and other such foods. To occasionally indulge is permissible; however, to regularly consume foods high in sugar and empty-calories (candy, soft drinks, cakes) is not recommended.

Eating Four or Five Times Daily

In order to eat all the foods previously recommended daily, a mother should eat more often by adding some sensible snacks made up of milk products and fresh or even dried fruit.

Digestion is thus facilitated, absorption is improved, and the quantities consumed at mealtime remain at a reasonable level. Small snacks are a source of energy, which enable a mother to take well-deserved pauses and rest periods during the day.

Problem Foods or Fluids

In reality, very few foods or fluids can seriously harm the mother or the child during the lactation period. However:
- Some may cause digestive problems in the nursing mother such as fried foods and foods which are too rich or too sweet, but these, in any case, are hardly advisable for anyone.
- Strong-tasting vegetables such as cabbage, onions, or garlic can alter the taste of breast-milk, but few babies object to this variation. It is better to experiment and see how a baby reacts to these vegetables rather than to completely eliminate them.
- Very spicy and salty foods also alter the taste of breast-milk. However, generally speaking, no one should overindulge in these foods, least of all nursing mothers.
- Chocolate's deservedly bad reputation is probably valid since certain unfortunate reactions have been noticed in babies whose mothers ate chocolate in large amounts (constipation, eczema, irritability, wakefulness). Here, as elsewhere, the "quantity and frequency" factor should be considered. It is not the occasional small piece of chocolate which is to blame, but rather the daily chocolate bar and the regular eating of other chocolate or cocoa products.
- Fresh-water fish (yellow pike, pike, trout, bass), especially from the contaminated water of the St. Lawrence River, its tributaries, or neighboring lakes, is not recommended for nursing mothers since they often contain high levels of PCBs (polychlorated biphenyls). Seafoods (cod, sole, haddock, halibut) do not present any problem and can be eaten liberally and frequently by the nursing mother.
- Coffee and tea stimulate the mother and can over-

stimulate the baby if they are consumed in great amounts. Moderation is beneficial in many situations, for both mother and child.

- Alcohol is rapidly assimilated in breast-milk and can harm the baby if consumed in large quantities. On the other hand, the "occasional" glass of wine or beer is often recommended by pediatricians as a source of relaxation and fluid consumption for the mother.

Supplements: Essential or Superfluous?

As stated in the chapter about pregnancy, a nursing mother does not, in principle, require vitamin or mineral supplements. But, in actual fact, a high percentage of nursing mothers continues to use prenatal supplements during the nursing period.

When the effect of taking these supplements is evaluated, with regard to the nutrient composition of the breast-milk and the maternal reserves of well-nourished mothers, there is no appreciable difference between mothers who take supplements and those who do not. It should be remembered that we are discussing properly-fed mothers — the solution rests in what a mother eats!

- If a mother does not drink at least two large glasses of milk per day, a daily supplement of 200 IU (international units) of vitamin D in liquid or tablet form is necessary in order to make full use of the calcium found in the cheese or yogurt eaten daily. (Liquid milk is the only milk product enriched with vitamin D in Canada and the total daily requirement is obtained by drinking 500 mL (16 oz.). Other milk products are not vitamin D enriched. In the U.S., enrichment of milk with vitamin D is optional.)
- If a mother does not incorporate a sufficient amount of milk products in her diet, that is, the equivalent of a litre (1 quart) of milk in the form of cheese, yogurt, or milk-based dishes, she must add a calcium supplement in order to reach 1,200 mg of calcium per day. Otherwise she will lose calcium from her own bones.

- If a mother is a "strict vegetarian," that is, she does not eat any meat, milk products, or eggs, she should take supplements of vitamin B12, calcium, and vitamin D in order not to damage a baby's growth or development.

  Daily needs:
  2.5 Ug of vitamin B12 (4 Ug in U.S.)
  1,200 mg of calcium (1,200 mg in U.S.)
  200 IU of vitamin D (400 IU in U.S.)*

- If the mother's diet is definitely insufficient, she should continue the daily use of prenatal supplements until her diet improves!

Pay Close Attention to Using Medication!

The baby receives, in spite of himself, everything that a mother eats: food, liquids, medication, or drugs. A magic filter which allows only the good substances to enter the mammary glands from the maternal blood does not exist. Everything is transmitted to the baby and can affect his incomplete digestive and renal system.

All medication taken by the mother is thus passed in small amounts into the breast-milk. Most have little effect on the child, but some, such as anticoagulants, hypothyroids, amphetamines, and diuretics, must be avoided. The use of the birth-control pill during the lactation period is still quite controversial since it reduces the quantity of the breast-milk and leaves traces of hormones. If absolutely necessary, a minimal dose prescribed by a consulting physician, and containing progesterone only, seems preferable.

As a general guideline concerning medication, abstinence is desirable when possible. In case of necessity, a treating physician should be consulted.

---

*Note: The amounts of nutrients suggested by the "Recommended Nutrient Intakes for Canadians" (1982) may slightly differ from the ones put forward by the U.S. "Recommended Dietary Allowances" (1980); these variations reflect the consensus reached by two different committees of experts and should not detract from the purpose of the recommendations; the requirements should be considered as levels of intake that can maintain health of the majority of the "already" healthy population. This data also applies to Tables VI-1, XIII-2, XIII-3.

Menu-Planning Time!

In order to make use of the recommendations contained in this chapter, the following pages present seven complete menus for "carnivorous" nursing mothers, and seven complete menus adapted for "lacto-ovo vegetarian" nursing mothers. The nutritive value of the menus is then analyzed.

Menus for Nursing Mothers

With Meat

DAY 1

BREAKFAST
½ grapefruit
banana bread with ricotta or cottage cheese (¼ cup or 60 mL)
glass of milk or café au lait (8 oz. or 250 mL)

LUNCH
raw vegetables
lentil soup (1 cup or 250 mL)
whole-wheat bread (2 slices)
plain yogurt with fresh or canned peaches (4 oz. or 125 mL)
fruit and milk (8 oz. or 250 mL)

DINNER
baked chicken (3 oz. or 90 gm)
orange rice
carrots and green beans
baked apple
herbal tea
milk or yogurt (8 oz. or 250 mL)

DAY 2
BREAKFAST
orange juice

Vegetarian

DAY 1

BREAKFAST
½ grapefruit
banana bread with ricotta or cottage cheese (¼ cup or 60 mL)
glass of milk or café au lait (8 oz. or 250 mL)

LUNCH
raw vegetables
lentil soup (1 cup or 250 mL)
whole-wheat bread (2 slices)
plain yogurt with fresh or canned peaches (4 oz. or 125 mL)
fruit and milk (8 oz. or 250 mL)

DINNER
oven-baked vegetable casserole
herb bread
salad greens
baked apple
herbal tea
milk or yogurt (8 oz. or 250 mL)

DAY 2
BREAKFAST
orange juice

oatmeal with raisins and milk
whole-wheat bread, toasted
 (1 slice)
milk or café au lait (6 oz. or
 180 mL)

LUNCH
raw vegetables
grilled salmon sandwich or pita
 bread stuffed with salmon
banana
glass of milk (8 oz. or 250 mL)

fruit juice and cheese (1½ oz.
 or 45 gm)

DINNER
lentil and brown-rice casserole
zucchini and carrots
gingerbread and orange
 yogurt (4 oz. or 125 mL)
herbal tea

milk or yogurt (8 oz.)

DAY 3
BREAKFAST
quartered orange
egg (hard-boiled or poached)
whole-wheat bread, toasted
 (2 slices)
milk or café au lait (8 oz. or
 250 mL)

LUNCH
salad of cooked and raw
 vegetables
cheese cubes (2 oz. or 60 gm)
 and nuts
slice of whole-wheat bread or
 bran muffin
fresh or canned pears
milk

milk and dried fruits (8 oz. or
 250 mL)

oatmeal with raisins and milk
whole-wheat bread, toasted
 (1 slice)
milk or café au lait (6 oz. or
 180 mL)

LUNCH
raw vegetables
one grilled English muffin
 spread with peanut butter or
 cheese
banana
glass of milk (8 oz. or 250 mL)
fruit juice and cheese (1½ oz.
 or 45 gm)

DINNER
lentil and brown-rice casserole
zucchini and carrots
gingerbread and orange
 yogurt (4 oz. or 125 mL)
herbal tea

milk or yogurt (8 oz. or 25 mL)

DAY 3
BREAKFAST
quartered orange
egg (hard-boiled or poached)
whole-wheat bread, toasted
 (2 slices)
milk or café au lait (8 oz. or
 250 mL)

LUNCH
salad of cooked and raw
 vegetables
cheese cubes (2 oz. or 60 gm)
 and nuts
slice of whole-wheat bread or
 bran muffin
fresh or canned pears
milk

milk and dried fruits (8 oz. or
 250 mL)

DINNER
pot roast (3 oz. or 90 gm)
coleslaw with apples
slice of whole-wheat bread
fresh fruit cocktail
herbal tea or water

milk or yogurt (8 oz. or
250 mL)

DAY 4
BREAKFAST
½ grapefruit
shredded wheat cereal with
milk garnished with nuts
and wheat germ
slice of whole-wheat bread,
toasted
milk or café au lait (6 oz. or
180 mL)

LUNCH
vegetable juice or soup
chopped egg sandwich (1 egg)
on slice of whole-wheat
bread
apple sauce
milk (8 oz. or 250 mL)

apple and cheese cube (1½ oz.
or 45 gm)

DINNER
poached fish fillet (4 oz. or
120 gm)
baked potato
plain broccoli
banana with yogurt sauce
(4 oz. or 125 mL)
herbal tea

milk or yogurt (8 oz. or
250 mL)

DINNER
red kidney beans (1 cup or
250 mL) with herbs and rice
(½ cup or 125 mL)
coleslaw with apples
slice of whole-wheat bread
fresh fruit cocktail
herbal tea or water

milk or yogurt (8 oz. or
250 mL)

DAY 4
BREAKFAST
½ grapefruit
shredded wheat cereal with
milk garnished with nuts
and wheat germ
slice of whole-wheat bread,
toasted
milk or café au lait (6 oz. or
180 mL)

LUNCH
vegetable juice or soup
chopped egg sandwich (1 egg)
on slice of whole-wheat
bread
apple sauce
milk (8 oz. or 250 mL)

apple and cheese cube (1½ oz.
or 45 gm)

DINNER
stuffed vegetable crêpes au
gratin
salad greens
banana with yogurt sauce
(4 oz. or 125 mL)
herbal tea

milk or yogurt (8 oz. or
250 mL)

DAY 5

BREAKFAST
orange juice
1 poached or hard-boiled egg
2 slices of whole-wheat bread,
   toasted
milk or café au lait (8 oz. or
   250 mL)

LUNCH
cream of green vegetable soup
Romaine lettuce salad with
   beans (1 cup)
2 slices whole-wheat bread
yogurt with fresh or canned
   peaches (4 oz. or 125 mL)
milk (8 oz. or 250 mL)

raisins and milk (8 oz. or
   250 mL)

DINNER
beef liver creole (3 oz. or
   90 gm)
brown rice with parsley (1 cup
   or 250 mL)
french green beans
apple sauce
herbal tea

milk or yogurt (8 oz. or
   250 mL)

DAY 6

BREAKFAST
apple juice
shredded wheat sprinkled with
   nuts, raisins and milk
1 slice whole-wheat bread
   toasted or 1 bran muffin
milk or café au lait (6 oz. or
   180 mL)

LUNCH
raw vegetables
grilled cheese (2 oz. or 60 gm)
   sandwich with tomato

DAY 5

BREAKFAST
orange juice
1 poached or hard-boiled egg
2 slices whole-wheat bread,
   toasted
milk or café au lait (8 oz. or
   250 mL)

LUNCH
cream of green vegetable soup
Romaine lettuce salad with
   beans (1 cup)
2 slices whole-wheat bread
yogurt with fresh or canned
   peaches (4 oz. or 125 mL)
milk (8 oz. or 250 mL)

raisins and milk (8 oz. or
   250 mL)

DINNER
vegetable juice
vegetable pizza with lots of
   cheese
chinese cabbage salad
apple sauce
herbal tea

milk or yogurt (8 oz. or
   250 mL)

DAY 6

BREAKFAST
apple juice
shredded wheat sprinkled with
   nuts, raisins and milk
1 slice whole-wheat bread
   toasted or 1 bran muffin
milk or café au lait (6 oz. or
   180 mL)

LUNCH
raw vegetables
grilled-cheese (2 oz. or 60 gm)
   sandwich with tomato

apple or pear
milk (8 oz. or 250 mL)

fruit and milk (4 oz. or 125 mL)

braised beef with parslied
 noodles
1 slice whole-wheat bread
lettuce-and-spinach salad
yogurt (4 oz. or 125 mL) and
 strawberries
herbal tea

milk (4 oz. or 125 mL)

DAY 7
BREAKFAST
quartered orange
1 oz. (30 gm) cheese
2 bran muffins
milk or café au lait (8 oz. or
 250 mL)

LUNCH
vegetable juice or broth
chicken and rice salad
1 slice whole-wheat bread
banana with yogurt sauce
 (4 oz. or 125 mL)
milk (8 oz. or 250 mL)

raisins and nuts
milk (8 oz. or 250 mL)

DINNER
cheese omelette (2 eggs)
chinese cabbage salad
2 slices whole-wheat bread
baked apple
oatmeal cookie (1)
herbal tea

milk or yogurt (4 oz. or
 125 mL)

apple or pear
milk (8 oz. or 250 mL)

fruit and milk (4 oz. or 125 mL)

DINNER
baked beans à la québécoise
 with parslied rice
1 slice whole-wheat bread
lettuce-and-spinach salad
yogurt (4 oz. or 125 mL) and
 strawberries
herbal tea

milk (4 oz. or 125 mL)

DAY 7
BREAKFAST
quartered orange
1 oz. (30 gm) cheese
2 bran muffins
milk or café au lait (8 oz. or
 250 mL)

LUNCH
raw vegetables
lentil or pea soup (1 cup or
 250 mL)
2 slices whole-wheat bread
banana and yogurt sauce
 (4 oz. or 125 mL)
milk (8 oz. or 250 mL)

raisins and nuts
milk (8 oz. or 250 mL)

DINNER
cheese omelette (2 eggs)
chinese cabbage salad
2 slices whole-wheat bread
baked apple
oatmeal cookie (1)
herbal tea

milk or yogurt (4 oz. or
 125 mL)

VI-1: *Nutritive Values of the 7 Menus for Nursing Mothers*

A. Meat Menus (4 to 4½ oz. (125-135 gm) of poultry, meat, or fish per day)

Menus	Calories	Protein (g)	Calcium (mg)	Iron (mg)	Vit. B12 (Ug)	Vit. C (mg)
Day 1	1985	104	1556	16	5	213
Day 2	2415	97	2119	15	10	251
Day 3	2367	104	2074	17	10	322
Day 4	1800	102	1858	14	7	159
Day 5	2192	114	2253	22[3]	78[3]	297
Day 6	2138	95	1968	18	6	219
Day 7	2194	105	2020	18	7	193
DAILY AVERAGE	2156[1]	103[2]	1978	17	18	236[4]
Quantities Recommended:						
Canada	2400-2600	61	1200	14	2.5	75
U.S.A.	2500-2600	64	1200	30-60[5]	4	100

1. The average caloric content is below that recommended by the Recommended Nutrient Intakes for Canadians and the Recommended Dietary Allowances (U.S.) but approaches the actual quantities consumed by nursing mothers. Furthermore, the amounts shown do not include the fats normally used in cooking and as spreads, except those used for dressings. In most cases, 2% milk and plain yogurt are used.It would, therefore, be easy to adjust the calories contained in this diet if so desired.
2. Regardless of the fact that the meat, poultry, and fish portions are small, the menus contain much more protein than recommended.
3. Day 5 menu is very rich in iron and vitamin B12 because it contains liver, a super-rich food in both these nutrients.
4. A high amount of vitamin C contained in these diets reflects a high fruit and vegetable content. This also implies that vitamin supplements are unnecessary when one eats properly.
5. Iron needs during lactation are not substantially different from those of non-pregnant women, but con-

tinued supplementation of the mother for two to three months after birth is sometimes advised in order to replenish stores depleted by pregnancy.

B. *Vegetarian Menus (without meat, but containing milk products and eggs)*

Menus	Calories	Protein (g)	Calcium (mg)	Iron (mg)	Vit. B12 (Ug)	Vit. C (mg)
Day 1	1914	86	1857	15	5	168
Day 2	2361	86	1952	14	4	251
Day 3	2331	98	2300	18	9	373
Day 4	2018	96	2336	16	7	184
Day 5	2164	99	2423	15	12	284
Day 6	2076	84	2078	20	4	258
Day 7	2129	95	2067	17	6	144
DAILY AVERAGE	2142[1]	92	2145	16[3]	7[4]	237
Canada	2400-2600	66[2]	1200	14	2.5	75
U.S.A.	2500-2600	64	1200	30-60[5]	4	100

1. Comments about the caloric values of these vegetarian menus are the same as those made about the meat diet.
2. The protein recommendation of 66 grams per day in a vegetarian diet represents an 8% increase over that of the meat diet and meets the FAO's recommendations in this respect. According to the same source, a "vegan" diet without meat, milk products, or eggs would require a daily addition of 13 grams of protein; that is, an increase of 21% in relation to the meat diet, to make up for the total absence of food of animal origin.
3. Due to daily consumption of whole-grain cereals and legumes, the average iron values slightly exceed the Canadian recommendation of 14 grams per day. However, it is important to realize that iron, from these sources, is not used as efficiently by the body as the iron from meat or organ meats. If a vitamin-C rich fruit or vegetable is eaten (orange, broccoli, or other) at mealtime, together with legumes or cereal, iron is absorbed five times more efficiently than if these foods were eaten alone.

4. Adequate amounts of vitamin B12 are found in vegetarian diets since they contain large amounts of milk products and eggs. A "vegan" diet without meat, poultry, fish, milk products or eggs will not contain enough vitamin B12 and could have serious effects on the mother unless vitamin B12 supplements are added or she adjusts her diet accordingly.
5. Iron needs during lactation are not substantially different from those of non-pregnant women, but continued supplementation for two or three months after birth is sometimes advised in order to replenish stores depleted during pregnancy.

CHAPTER SEVEN

"Other Milks" Before and After Six Months

DURING THE FIRST YEAR of life, breast-milk or another carefully chosen milk continues to be the most important baby food and is unequalled in supplying important nutritive elements necessary to the baby's growth. No other food can do as much! During the first six months, milk alone suffices. After this age, solids complete the picture, milk still retaining its principal role.

Many chapters of this book expound upon the benefits of breast-feeding because it is the first and best choice. Unfortunately, at the present time, only a relatively small number of babies (50% in the U.S., 48% in France) benefit from it and only for a short period of one to sixteen weeks. A vast assortment of milks is thus consumed by babies, and various surveys conducted in Canada and the U.S. reveal the breakdown of these milks during the first months.

VII-1: Other Types of Milk Found in a Baby's Diet

Other types of milk	% of babies drinking at birth	% of babies drinking before 6 months
"Humanized" formulas (SMA, Similac, Enfalac)	50 to 77	31
Cow's milk, homogenized, whole	0.3 to 12	52
2% or skim	2 to 8	10.5

As the table shows, all babies do not drink the same type of milk at birth, and a large number of them change to another milk before they are six months old. Some breast-fed babies at birth also change to other types of milk before the age of six months. As well, one-third of all babies, regardless of the mode of feeding, drink three types of milk during the first year of life.

Some milks are definitely unsuitable choices to use at birth since they can harm the newborn's organism, such as ordinary cow's milk, 2%, 1% or skim; while others, such as "humanized" formulas, are recommended. After six months the situation changes, and whole cow's milk can be given without any problem.

In order to provide the baby with the right milk at the right time, let us examine the composition and nutritive value of these various milks. Let it be well understood, however, the final choice should be made in consultation with the doctor. The following humanized formulas are recommended for the first six months failing breast-feeding:

- in Canada and in the United States: SMA, Similac, Enfalac, PM 60/40, Enfamil
- in Europe: Aptamil, Lacmil, Materna Spécial, Nan, Nativa, Nidina Maternisé, Nursie, S26.

Although these milks attempt to imitate breast-milk as much as possible, they cannot, because breast-milk is inimitable. One need only observe the periodic changes made to the composition of these milks and the variations from one milk to the other which follow upon the heels of the most recent discoveries in breast-milk research and recommendations from leading experts in the field.

Nevertheless, on the whole these milks are more suitable to the physiological needs of the newborn than ordinary cow's milk or other available milks; they are the second-best choice after breast-milk.

Simulated Milks

1. Composition

Certain humanized milk formulas (Enfalac, Similac) are manufactured in the following way:

a) cow's milk is first skimmed, then diluted. This decreases the amount of protein and minerals, and the resulting concentrations then closely resemble the amounts found in breast-milk

b) vegetable oils (coconut oil, corn oil, soya oil) are then added to the milk to replace the fat found in cow's milk which the baby has more trouble digesting and which contains less polyunsaturated fats than some of the vegetable oils used as substitutes

c) lactose (milk sugar) is also added to equal the levels of lactose present in breast-milk. This type of sugar is preferable to all others, since once it is transformed into galactose, it is the only sugar capable of being used for building of the baby's brain cells.

Other humanized formulas (SMA and PM 60/40) are made up of equal quantities of skimmed cow's milk and "demineralized whey milk" which better simulates the amount of protein and minerals found in breast-milk. These formulas also contain vegetable oils in place of the fat in cow's milk and additional lactose in order to attain the same levels as those normally found in breast-milk.

Several of these humanized formulas are available with additional amounts of iron (SMA, iron-enriched Similac, iron-enriched Enfalac). A doctor should determine whether there is a need to use an iron-enriched formula.

2. Nutritive Value

If humanized milk formulas are compared to ordinary cow's milk, the nutritive differences which affect the newborn's well-being are quickly understood.

VII-2: Table Comparing Humanized Milk Formulas and Cow's Milk

Nutritive Elements	Humanized Milk (SMA, Similac, Enfalac)	Cow's Milk (whole, homogenized)
Proteins	1.5 g/100 mL • quantity comparable to that found in breast-milk	3.5 g/100 mL • quantity exceeding the needs of the newborn

	• easier to digest since the milk is treated	• hard to digest by the baby
Fats	3.6 g/100 mL • vegetable oils (coconut, corn, soya) easier to digest and richer in polyunsaturated fats	3.5 g/100 mL • harder to digest and contains fewer polyunsaturated fats
Sugar	7.2 g/100 mL • lactose • useful to baby and found in amounts comparable to that found in breast-milk	4.9 g/100 mL • lactose • useful sugar for baby, but present in insufficient amounts
Minerals (calcium, phosphorous, potassium magnesium, etc.)	• found in lesser amounts than in cow's milk; comparable to amounts found in breast-milk	• greatly exceeds the baby's needs and his immature renal system is subjected to additional strain
Vitamin C	5.3 mg/100 mL • amount added is slightly above that present in breast-milk	1 mg/100 mL • amount insufficient to meet needs of baby
Vitamin D	42 IU/100 mL • amount added equals that found in cow's milk • compulsory enrichment in Canada	40 IU/100 mL • amount added in Canada to meet the high needs of children • enrichment compulsory in Canada, optional in the U.S.

3. Directions for Using Formulas

Humanized formulas should be prepared according to the instructions on the package, but keep these points in mind:

- while preparing the milk, use only scrupulously clean utensils which have been rinsed in boiling water
- sugar should never be added, as humanized milk contains the proper amount of sugar
- the milk formula is kept in sterilized bottles in the refrigerator until feeding time
- if the product is bought in "concentrated liquid" form, an equal amount of water is added (tap water must be boiled for twenty minutes, then cooled). If using "bottled" water, only those labelled "sterile" should be used and should not contain a large amount of mineral salts. These recommended products which meet these requirements include Canaqua, Evian, Labrador, Polar Spring pure natural mineral water, and Mountain Valley
- if the product is bought in "powdered" form, the correct amount of water and powder is measured out precisely to obtain the mixture suited to the baby's needs
- when the ready-to-serve type is used, shake the container before opening, and open and empty the desired amount into a sterilized baby bottle. Once opened, the can should be covered and refrigerated, and any unused amount should be discarded after forty-eight hours.

4. Time of Introduction and Length of Use

For previously mentioned reasons, humanized milk formulas are offered right at birth. They can occasionally be used to replace a breast-feeding or become a substitute for breast-feeding as in the case of early weaning.

Apart from breast-milk these are the only milks really suitable to the needs of infants less than six months old. After six months, the baby can gradually be changed from humanized formulas to whole cow's milk (3.25% fat).

5. Cost

Humanized formulas are available in drug stores and food stores. Prices vary enormously from one store to the next.

It would therefore be wise to visit several stores before buying a large quantity. Note: Bought in "powdered" form, the cost is half the cost of the ready-to-serve liquid form. Consult the table of daily cost comparisons found in Chapter Four.

Whole Homogenized Cow's Milk

Not recommended before six months

As you can very well see for yourself in Table VII-2, whole homogenized cow's milk is not at all suited to the needs of the newborn.

A baby should not drink this type of milk before six months of age. Whole cow's milk contains hard-to-digest protein and fats as well as too large a quantity of minerals which puts a strain on the baby's immature renal system. Occasionally, it can provoke allergic reactions, intestinal bleeding, and diarrhea accompanied by fever which can dehydrate the baby.

Note: If for reasons of serious budget problems, it becomes impossible to buy expensive humanized formulas, concentrated or evaporated whole cow's milk (3.25% fat: Carnation, Crino, Farmer's Wife) could become a third acceptable choice for the baby as long as it is reconstituted, diluted, and sweetened according to the doctor's or a health professional's directions (make sure Vitamin D is added if bought in the United States). The evaporation process alters cow's milk to some extent, and makes it more tolerable for the young baby. Concentrated or "evaporated" whole milk thus causes fewer intestinal problems than "untreated" milk.

No problem after six months

After six months, and once the baby has started eating solids, whole cow's milk containing 3.25% fat can gradually be integrated into his milk diet.

2%, 1% and Skim Milk

Not recommended during the first twelve months

Since the beginning of the '70s, it has been noticed that a growing number of babies have been drinking skim or 2% milk since birth or from four to six months onwards and under the pretext that this will alleviate problems of atherosclerosis or prevent obesity. In good faith at that time, we even suggested the 2% milk option in the first edition of this book.

A few researchers eager to discover the effects of this practice on the child's growth conducted a study on the question. They found that babies given skim milk from the age of four months drank larger amounts of milk and ate more solid foods than babies given humanized milk in order to obtain the needed energy essential for their growth. In spite of this, the former gained weight less rapidly and lost an important amount of fatty tissue, representing nearly 28% of their reserves over a fifty-six-day period as compared to the latter group. This considerable loss of fatty tissue could jeopardize the baby's ability to fight against infections or prolonged illness.

According to the authors, this type of milk, if given too early to the child, instead of preventing obesity seems to trigger a compensatory mechanism making him eat and drink larger quantities of food and milk in an attempt to obtain the desired satiety level. At an older age, faced with a diet richer in calories and fat, the child is unable to limit himself to moderate quantities, since he has acquired the habit of gorging himself to satisfy his appetite, and all this as a result of a too early introduction to skim milk.

It is also obvious that a 2%, 1% or skim-milk diet causes even greater harm in the newborn since it deprives the baby of essential fats normally contained in good quantities in breast-milk or humanized milk and in lesser amounts in whole cow's milk.

Two percent and skim milks also provide too much protein and minerals and tax the baby's immature, under-developed renal system. They are "unbalanced" milks for the newborn as well as all babies up to one year of age and should be avoided at all costs.

Soya or Meat-Based Formulas for "Special Cases"

It is possible to obtain a wide variety of other milk formulas based either on meat protein (HSC Lambs base, MBF) or soya protein (Prosobee, Isomil, Neo-Mull-Soy, etc.).

These formulas are used only in special cases, notably when babies are diagnosed "allergic" to the protein and/or the sugar (lactose) in milk. The baby's physician should be the only one who decides on the use of these formulas.

VII-3: *The Right Milk at the Right Time*

Milk	Introduction Time	Length of Use
Breast-milk	birth	unlimited, according to the mother's availability
Humanized milk formulas	birth	at least to the age of six months
Whole cow's milk	after 6 months and introduction of solids	until age 1 or older (according to family practices)
2% milk	after 1 year	according to the needs and food habits of the family
Skim milk	if necessary only after 12 months	according to the needs of the child

CHAPTER EIGHT

Vitamin Supplements
Before and After Six Months

WHEN ONE SPEAKS of vitamin or mineral supplements, essentially what is meant is a nutritional "complement"; the role of this "complement" is not to help the baby exceed his nutritional needs but rather to provide him with those nutrients which are not present in his daily diet in sufficient amounts. A vitamin or mineral supplement is useful, therefore, to "complete" the daily diet or to fill nutritional gaps which result when the foods consumed in a day do not provide all the nutritional needs of the baby.

In North America, the role of supplements is apparently misunderstood since a large majority of babies receives supplements automatically when they leave the hospital. The thinking behind this must be "more is better"! It must be admitted, vitamins in a prescribed dose cannot harm a baby or a young child. The use of these supplements from the second week of life as standard practice is debatable, nonetheless.

Opinions regarding the use of these supplements is divided, and often even contradictory. This book is not aimed at settling the debate once and for all, as a book can never replace the advice of a medical professional regarding the particular needs of a baby. The following pages present the facts and invite reflection. Before investing in expensive vitamin and mineral supplements, it is advisable to discuss them with your family physician.

The First Six Months

By drawing a parallel between the prescribed supplements, the needs of the baby, and his daily diet, it should be easy to determine if supplements are necessary. Unfortunately, this type of comparison would show only one side of the coin, since the infant has other sources of nutrients! Under ideal conditions, an infant is born with built-in nutrients assimilated during the gestation period and delivery. Borne by a well-nourished mother, and beneficiary of the placental transfusion at delivery prior to cutting the umbilical cord, the baby has had at its disposal nutritional reserves which are difficult to quantify, but are nevertheless real. There is no need to rearrange his nutritional requirements by altering his daily diet for merely a question of milligrams. Only wide variances should be supplemented and even then there are many exceptions!

To better understand the debate, let us begin by examining the daily contribution of various milks compared to the needs of the baby as estimated in the Recommended Nutrient Intakes for Canadians and the Recommended Dietary Allowances in the U.S. Then, we will look at the contribution of the most frequently prescribed supplements and draw the proper conclusions. Each nutritive element is studied separately and calculations are based on two volumes of milk, 800 mL and 1 litre (26 ounces and 31 ounces) in order to take into consideration the increase in the baby's milk consumption from birth to six months.

Vitamin D

Vitamin D is found in sufficient quantities in humanized milk and in concentrated milk (see Table VIII-1). (Vitamin D enrichment of concentrated milks is optional in the U.S.) On the other hand, only traces are found in human milk. In human milk, it is found in very small quantities and it cannot always prevent rickets among totally breast-fed babies. For this reason, a vitamin-D supplement is recommended for the breast-fed baby.

Since supplements containing only vitamin D are practically nonexistent, a supplement such as "Tri-vi-sol" is recommended for breast-fed babies beginning in the second week of life.

Babies fed the other types of recommended milks (see Chapter Seven) do not require any vitamin D supplement whatsoever.

VIII-1: *Daily Sources of Vitamin D before 6 Months*

Daily Diet	Daily Contribution	
	800 mL (26 oz.)	**1 litre (31 oz.)**
Human milk	30 IU	40 IU
Humanized milk (Enfalac, Similac, SMA)	320 IU	400 IU
Concentrated milk (Carnation or Crino, sweetened, evaporated, diluted, vitamin-D enriched)	380 IU	470 IU
Infant's requirements	400 IU/day	
Supplement:		
Tri-vi-sol	400 IU in 0.6 mL (recommended dosage in Canada)	
Tri-vi-sol Infant Drops	400 IU in 1.0 mL (in U.S.A.)	
Tri-vi-flor	200 IU in 0.3 mL (recommended dosage in Canada)	
Tri-vi-flor Infant Drops	400 IU in 1.0 mL (in U.S.A.)	

Vitamin C

Vitamin C is present in sufficient quantities in all milks recommended for babies. A supplement is therefore not necessary.

On the other hand, a baby fed cow's milk (an unrecommended milk) requires a vitamin-C supplement.

Breast-fed babies who are given a vitamin supplement containing three vitamins in order to obtain their quota of vitamin D, could perhaps benefit from vitamin C as it promotes better absorption of the iron found in breast-milk.

VIII-2: *Daily Sources of Vitamin C before 6 Months*

Daily Diet	Daily Contribution	
	800 mL (26 oz.)	1 litre (31 oz.)
Human milk	34 mg	43 mg
Humanized milk (Enfalac, Similac, SMA)	44 mg	55 mg
Whole concentrated milk (Carnation, Crino, evaporated, diluted and sweetened)	65 mg	80 mg
Infant's requirements	20 mg/day Canada 35 mg/day U.S.	
Supplement: Tri-vi-sol	30 mg in 0.6 mL (recommended dosage in Canada)	
Tri-vi-sol Infant Drops	35 mg in 1.0 mL (in U.S.A.)	
Tri-vi-flor	15 mg in 0.3 mL recommended dosage	
Tri-vi-flor Infant Drops	35 mg in 1.0 mL (in U.S.A.)	

Vitamin A

The baby's vitamin A requirements are satisfactorily met by his milk diet regardless of the type of milk used (Table VIII-3). The supplement simply provides a nonessential additional amount which, if administered in the proper dosage, does not harm the baby. We could ask ourselves why this vitamin continues to be present in these supplements when it rarely corresponds to a real deficiency in the baby's diet.

VIII-3: *Daily Sources of Vitamin A before 6 Months*

Daily Diet	Daily Contribution	
	800 mL (26 oz.)	1 litre (31 oz.)
Human milk	1600 IU	2000 IU
Humanized milk (Enfalac, Similac, SMA)	2000 IU	2500 IU
Whole concentrated milk (Carnation, Crino evaporated, diluted and sweetened, vitamin A enriched)	2000 IU	2400 IU
Infant's requirements	1400 IU/day	
Supplement: Tri-vi-sol	2500 IU in 0.6 mL (recommended dosage in Canada)	
Tri-vi-sol Infant Drops	1500 IU in 1.0 mL (U.S.A.)	
Tri-vi-flor	1250 IU in 0.3 mL (recommended dosage in Canada)	
Tri-vi-flor Infant Drops	1500 IU in 1.0 mL (in U.S.A.)	

B Vitamins

Some supplements (Ostoco, Infantol) contain vitamins from the B-complex (thiamin, riboflavin, niacin and vitamin B6) as well as vitamins A, D, and C. These vitamins are rarely necessary because breast-milk, humanized milk, or whole concentrated milk, diluted and sweetened, contain sufficient amounts these vitamins.

In a few cases, an additional quantity of B vitamins could

be required for the baby who drinks soya-based milk because of milk allergies. In such cases, the family doctor is your best guide.

Fluoride

Despite its rather controversial reputation, fluoride is a particularly important nutrient during the formative years. It has a marked effect on tooth formation, and many painful moments spent in the dentist's chair are avoided because fluoride helps form tooth enamel which is more resistant to various decay-producing agents. It has been found that regular drinking of fluoridated water helps reduce tooth decay by as much as 50% to 60%.

Since natural fluoride in food is quite limited, water fluoridation remains the best method of providing this nutrient to the population. The latest figures from the Center for Disease in Atlanta show that out of the 213 million people served by public water supplies in the U.S., nearly 106 million are now receiving fluoridated water. In all the United States about one half of the total population (46%) is receiving fluoridated water. From Western Europe there have been reports on remarkable reductions in tooth decay after fifteen years of water fluoridation in the Netherlands. By the time of the 25th anniversary of water fluoridation in the United States and Canada, there were over thirty countries around the world which had begun to implement this public health measure.

Until such time as all drinking water is fluoridated, babies in unfluoridated regions should receive a fluoride supplement after six months. Fluoride is effective mainly at teething time, and the supplement appears to be un-necessary and unbeneficial before a baby is six months old. Since it is often prescribed along with other vitamins at two weeks of age, a baby could feasibly take fluoride supplements from the second week following birth without danger.

A supplement such as "Karidium" contains fluoride exclusively, and a daily dose of two drops (0.25 mg) satisfies a baby's needs before or after six months.

Iron is part of the nutritional package received at birth. As all packages differ, this one, stored up during the last three months of pregnancy, is not equal in all newborn babies. A normal-weight baby born at term, who has a placental transfusion before the umbilical cord is cut, has good iron reserve for the next four months. A premature baby born at seven or eight months has generally exhausted all his iron reserves in two months. Babies cannot all be treated in the same way.

A baby also receives iron from the milk he drinks:

- Breast-milk contains little iron but is absorbed five times more efficiently than ordinary cow's milk or unenriched humanized milk. For this reason, breast-milk satisfies the baby's iron requirements entirely for at least six months without adding solid foods to his diet.
- Humanized unenriched milk (Enfalac, Similac) provides little iron, but can meet the iron needs of a normal-weight infant born at term for up to four months of age. When humanized milk is enriched with iron (Enfalac plus iron, Similac plus iron, or SMA), it satisfies a baby's requirements until the milk diet is altered.
- Whole concentrated milk (Crino, Carnation), diluted and sweetened, contains little iron, but does meet the requirements of a normal-weight infant born at term for up to four months of age.

In conclusion, as a general rule:

1. A normal-weight baby fed exclusively breast-milk for six months, without adding solids, does not need iron supplements until six months of age.

2. A normal-weight baby, fed iron-enriched humanized milk (Enfalac plus iron, Similac plus iron, or SMA) to six months of age, does not require the addition of iron supplements to his diet.

3. A normal-weight baby, fed ordinary humanized milk (Similac, Enfalac), or concentrated whole milk (Crino, Carnation, diluted and sweetened), needs additional iron

around four months. If this baby starts eating iron-enriched cereals around this time, he does not need any additional supplements. If he does not, 0.3 mL of Fer-in-Sol will supply him with 7.5 mg of iron per day. (Tri-vi-flor Infant Drops with iron supply 10 mg of iron in 1.0 mL.)

VIII-4: *Supplement Requirements for the Normal-Weight Baby, Born at Term, During the First 6 Months*

Nutritive Element	Maternal Milk	Humanized Milk (Similac, Enfalac)	Humanized Milk Iron-Enriched (Similac + iron, Enfalac + iron, SMA)	Concentrated Whole Milk (Crino, Carnation)
Vitamin D	supplement necessary at two weeks 400 IU/day	unnecessary	unnecessary	unnecessary
Vitamin C	unnecessary	unnecessary	unnecessary	unnecessary
Vitamin A	unnecessary	unnecessary	unnecessary	unnecessary
Fluoride	unnecessary	unnecessary	unnecessary	unnecessary
Iron	unnecessary	supplement necessary after 4 months (5-10 mg/day or iron-enriched baby cereals)	unnecessary	supplement necessary after 4 months (5-10 mg/day or iron-enriched baby cereals)

There is no general rule for underweight or premature babies. Your doctor should be consulted.

Six to Eighteen Months

A mother who gradually adds iron-enriched baby cereals, vegetables, poultry, fish or meat (legumes if vegetarian), and fruit to the baby's diet, sees that he receives all the required nutrients, provided a good supply of milk continues to be consumed. Such babies do not need vitamin or mineral supplements except fluoride if the municipality where the baby lives does not add it to the drinking water. In this case, 0.25 mg of fluoride is given in the form of "Karidium" drops represents the daily dose recommended up to age two.

Should a baby constantly refuse to eat one or more important food groups, a supplement should be added to his diet:

- the child who drinks only a small amount of milk or does not eat dairy products needs a supplement of calcium, vitamin D, and B vitamins
- the vegan child who does not eat eggs, milk, milk products, meat, poultry, or fish needs a vitamin D plus calcium and B12 supplement
- the child who constantly refuses to eat any fruit or vegetables benefits by taking vitamin A and C supplements (see Chapter Eleven for role and daily require ments of these vitamins from birth to six years).

CHAPTER NINE

Solid Foods: Slowly but Surely!

EARLY IN THIS century the infant ate no solid food before the age of one. This was the era of the fat, "milk-fed" baby! According to an extensive survey conducted in Montreal in 1976, 40% of babies were eating cereals by the age of two weeks, and one out of every two babies was receiving meat by three and one-half months. This was the era of the "forced-fed" baby.

This premature introduction to solid foods reflects the type of advice once given by certain doctors since very few mothers will on their own alter their baby's diet. However, two years ago, two surveys conducted among 1,000 doctors in British Columbia and Nebraska found that 44% to 81% of them recommended that solids not be introduced before the baby had reached the age of two months. And a recent and extensive study of the eating habits of over 400 babies in the Montreal and Toronto areas shows that the majority of babies surveyed are not being fed solids until they reach two months of age. This is a good step in the right direction!

Infant nutrition experts on the nutrition committee of the Canadian Pediatric Society, nutritionists from Canada, the United States, and Europe, and officials from various government bodies, are unanimous in saying that there are no advantages to be gained by introducing solids to babies before the age of four to six months.

Physiological, Nutritive and Anti-Allergenic Reasons for Introducing Solids after Four to Six Months of Age

The opinions and advice given by health professionals today is fairly consistent although some may vary by a few weeks, more or less, but the underlying message remains the same: "Before four to six months, a breast-fed baby receiving a vitamin D supplement, or a baby on a humanized milk formula, receives all the nourishment he needs."

This recommendation is based on arguments which are difficult to refute!

A. Solids have no effect on the length of the baby's sleep periods

Controlled scientific observations demonstrate that no relationship exists between the introduction of solid foods and the number of hours of nocturnal sleep a baby will have under four months of age. Many babies fed milk exclusively sleep all night long before four months. Prolonged sleep represents a baby's neurological development and has nothing to do with his eating habits.

B. Before a certain age, a baby is not physically ready to swallow solids

Before three months of age, a baby does not salivate very much, and his tongue is not able to push the food towards the back of his mouth. His "suction" reflex is well developed but his "ingurgitation" reflex is not; he has great trouble swallowing foods of a solid consistency. The neuromuscular coordination which enables him to eat solid foods adequately is reached around sixteen to eighteen weeks.

C. The newborn's digestive system is underdeveloped

At birth a baby is not equipped with all the "digestive apparatus" essential for the digestion of many foods. A full-term baby has only a fraction of the digestive enzymes or substances normally available in the six-month or two-year-old child. Before he has reached the age of three or four months, he is not ready to digest cereals or other starches and, before four to six months, he absorbs only part of the fats. A baby who eats solids too early only partially assimilates them and does so with great difficulty; what remains is found in his stools.

D. A baby's renal system is immature

The newborn infant is not really completely developed; his renal system is incomplete and very vulnerable to food excesses. Some foods, if given too early (meat, egg yolk), place a burden on the kidneys and may cause serious problems in more fragile babies or in babies drinking ordinary cow's milk during the first few months of life.

E. The younger the baby the higher the risks of allergic reactions

The immune defense system which protects the baby against hostile invaders is still incomplete in the four- to eight-week-old baby. The addition of solid food at this time could provoke an allergic reaction. The production of antibodies increases gradually during the first year, peaking at seven months. A slow and gradual introduction of solids after four to six months reduces the risks of allergic reactions particularly in babies whose families have a history of allergies.

F. A full-term baby does not require iron until four to six months

A full-term breast-fed baby given exclusively breast-milk does not require iron until he reaches the age of six months, while a baby fed humanized milk (not iron-enriched) uses up iron reserves by the time he is four months old. Baby cereals given between four to six months help meet increased dietary iron needs. Before that, their contribution is superfluous.

G. Early introduction of solid foods does not increase the nutritive value of the diet

In spite of his "immature" digestive, renal, and immunological development, the young baby does possess a satiety mechanism. For this reason when he is fed solid foods at too early an age, he automatically reduces his milk consumption.

In order to quantify this phenomenon properly, comparative studies have been carried out on the nutritive values of the diet of infants fed exclusively on milk and of the diet of those fed on milk and solids. The studies found that up to the age of three months the two diets were equal from the nutritional standpoint. The "milk and solid" diet is not superior because the baby is satisfied more quickly and drinks less milk. Solids replace milk, instead of complementing the milk, and are often (as in the case of cereals, fruits, and vegetables) less useful to the baby.

For the same number of calories, solids provide less of the important nutritive elements and may decrease the nutritive value of the entire diet of the baby.

H. The slow introduction of solids respects a baby's appetite

Around five or six months, a baby can easily sit up with support and has better neuromuscular control of his head and neck. He can reveal his hunger by moving his head forward and indicate his satiety by moving it back. Before a baby can do these movements or give these distinct messages, the feeding of solids is tantamount to force-feeding.

It is only possible to respect a baby's appetite, to foster good nutritive habits and prevent overeating when he can clearly indicate his hunger and his satisfaction. This final point is of prime importance to this author, and is a stepping-stone in forming good eating habits.

The Ideal Time for Introducing Solids

Between four to six months of age, a baby not only is able to swallow and digest a certain number of foods, but he also gradually acquires the capacity to chew solid food. He is also ready to experience new foods as far as texture and flavor are concerned. With half of his year behind him, the six-month-old baby is able to chew solid foods regardless of the fact that he does not have any teeth!

If the introduction of solids is delayed until nine or ten months, the value of this particularly sensitive and positive period could be lost. The older baby resists being fed foods of greater consistency, and to a change in his diet. It is more difficult for him to accept ordinary foods and he could "demand" strained baby food for a very long time!

Although everyone may agree on the ideal time for the introduction of solids, there is no universally perfect time for all babies. Each baby is different and should be treated as such. Few guidelines are available which can determine the precise and ideal time for a given baby. A baby's growth and general behavior are the best indicators to parents and to the family doctor.

- *The total amount of milk consumed during the day is not an absolute criteria!* Milk volume often varies from one baby to the next. A breast-fed baby drinks an unknown quantity of milk; a small baby at birth drinks less milk than a bigger one; the four- or five-month-old baby can easily drink about forty ounces of milk per day. In fact, no fixed rule exists which applies to all.

- *The number of feedings per day can sometimes be a poor indicator.* Up to four or five months of age, a baby drinks at least four times a day. If the number of feedings is reduced to three too quickly, a baby will have trouble drinking enough milk at each feeding. In such a situation, a baby demonstrating his hunger requires an additional milk feeding, and not solids.

- *Crying does not always indicate hunger.* Proper interpretation of the cries of a baby requires considerable parental intuition and sensitivity, and it is sometimes easier to attribute crying to hunger than to some other cause. By using the "milk or food" method as a last recourse, after eliminating other common sources of discomfort (dirty diapers, uncomfortable position, need for music and light, thirst), the various needs of the child are better respected and overfeeding is avoided.

Baby Cereals: A Necessity!

The argument for or against commercially prepared baby foods has somewhat tarnished the reputation of baby cereals. They have been accused of not meeting the nutritional needs of the infant and of containing sugar. However, if their nutritive contribution of protein, B vitamins and minerals is considered, these accusations appear unfounded!

Easily eaten and digested because they are precooked and reduced to a fine powder, these cereals are specially prepared to meet the needs of babies and to supply an important quantity of iron at a time when a baby's reserves are almost exhausted. These cereals are even preferable to oatmeal and other whole-grain cereals since they are enriched with a type of iron, particularly well suited to a baby's digestive system to a level based on the absorptive capacity of the baby's digestive system.

Reports from a recent survey of the food and nutrient intake of over 400 infants during their first eighteen months of life indicate that the iron intake of these infants was low from twelve months onward. Lack of adequate iron was attributed to early termination of iron-fortified infant cereals; many infants were eating adult-type cereals that were fortified with iron at a much lower level than the infant cereals.

Since they are nutritious and difficult to replace with ordinary cereals, it is sometimes recommended that they be included in a baby's diet up to eighteen months of age. The recommendation of the American Academy of Pediatrics is to include infant cereals in the diets of children up to two years of age.

It is true that while cereals containing sugar are still on the market, they are fewer and fewer in numbers. In 1977, manufacturers of baby foods in North America discontinued adding sugar to the majority of their cereals. Well-informed consumers can easily avoid buying "sweetened" cereals by reading the labels.

IX-1: *A Practical Guide to the Introduction of Cereals*

Time of introduction: between four and six months

Contribution:
- baby's iron reserves are nearly exhausted; cereals contribute good amounts of iron
- cereals provide iron, B vitamins, protein, and additional needed calories

Procedure:
- start with the cereals less likely to produce an allergic reaction (rice, barley, soya)
- begin with one teaspoon of cereal mixed with formula milk or breast-milk
- always spoon-feed in order to provide baby with exercise for the mouth muscles
- never add sugar
- serve the same cereal four or five days consecutively before introducing a new one
- gradually increase the amount to a maximum of eight tablespoons daily by the end of the first year
- cereals with fruit added are not recommended

Vegetables: A Way of Adding Color to the Diet

Vegetables should be added to the baby's diet, one month after starting cereals. They add color, texture, and flavor, and are more easily accepted if offered before fruit. They are also low in calories and add vitamins and food fiber to the newborn's diet.

Carrots are quite popular and are a good way to get things started! They should be followed by a variety of green, yellow, or white vegetables: green beans, zucchini, asparagus, green peas, broccoli, yellow beans, squash, and cauliflower.

Potatoes come last, around seven months, to complement the other vegetables and not to replace them.

IX-2: *A Practical Guide to the Introduction of Vegetables*

Time of introduction: one month after the introduction of cereals

Contribution:
- provide vitamins, minerals, and food fiber
- develop baby's taste buds

Procedure:
- introduce one vegetable at a time: wait four or five days before offering another one
- give each vegetable "separately" before offering a mixture of vegetables
- always give "cooked" vegetables
- use homemade purees or commercial baby food
- never add salt, sugar, or fat
- gradually increase the amount from 1 teaspoon to a maximum of 10 tablespoons toward the end of the first year
- always spoon-feed

Fruit for Dessert

Fruit stimulates a baby's taste buds and is easily integrated into his diet! Fruits supply vitamins, minerals, food fiber, and a permissible type of sugar. Apples, pears, bananas, peaches, and apricots form an interesting variety. Unsweetened fruit juice also provides vitamins, minerals and tastes good.

IX-3: *A Practical Guide to the Introduction of Fruit*

Time of introduction: three or four weeks after the introduction of vegetables

Contribution:
- vitamins, minerals, and food fiber
- flavor and permissible sugar

Procedure:
- offer each fruit "separately" before blending a mixture of fruit or fruit purees

- use homemade purees or commercial baby food
- offer "cooked" fruit except for ripe bananas which can simply be mashed with a fork
- small fruits such as strawberries, raspberries, gooseberries, and red grapes contain small seeds which may present some problems and should be avoided until the age of eighteen to twenty-four months
- never add sugar
- avoid fruit "desserts"
- to quench a baby's "thirst," water is preferable to repeated use of fruit juice.
- 2 oz. of fruit juice daily will meet all vitamin C needs

Meat, Poultry, Fish or Substitutes Complete the Menu

Providing important sources of protein, this food group is the last to be added to a baby's menu. Since the nutrients in meats and meat substitutes are more concentrated than in cereals, vegetables and fruit, they are better tolerated by the baby who is over six months of age.

Several fish, such as cod, haddock, sole, and boston blue fish, contain very little fat, have a delicate flavor, and provide protein of excellent quality.

Chicken liver is economical and nutritious, and can occasionally replace meat, providing an important amount of iron.

Cooked and mashed legumes or tofu (cheese made from the soya bean) contain good amounts of vegetable protein and can ensure normal growth for a vegetarian baby when adequately complemented in the diet.

One daily meat, poultry, or fish portion meets the nutritional needs of a baby.

IX-4: *A Practical Guide to the Introduction of Meat or Meat Substitutes*

Time of introduction: two to three weeks after the integration of fruit; this enables incorporation of only one food group at a time

Contribution:
- excellent source of protein
- meat, liver, and legumes rich in iron
- poultry and fish contain less fat than meat

Procedure:
- start with white meat (chicken, turkey) or fish
- use homemade purees or commercial baby food (pureed meat of one type only)
- at the start, do not mix with vegetables in order to encourage the distinguishing of different flavors
- never add salt
- gradually increase from a small amount to a maximum of 6 tablespoons daily toward the end of the first year
- the vegetarian baby can substitute cottage cheese, tofu, or cooked, pureed legumes for meat
- serve this food group preferably at the noon meal

Other Foods

Egg Yolk

Hardened and sifted in small quantities into pureed vegetables or meat, egg yolk is introduced into a baby's diet at the same time as meat or meat substitutes. It supplies protein, vitamins, and minerals, but is no longer considered a good source of iron.

One teaspoon (5 mL) per day is recommended at the beginning, preferably given at the noon meal, and it is gradually increased to a maximum of three egg yolks per week around twelve months of age. This food is not essential and can be eliminated from the diet in a "high risk" family; that is, a family with a history of high blood cholesterol levels.

Whole Egg

Since egg white causes more allergies than the yolk, the whole egg is introduced toward the end of the first year of life, when the baby's antibody system is better developed.

After one year, a poached or hard-boiled egg can be

served four times a week without any problems. As it is easily digested, it can be eaten at night surrounded by colorful vegetables. Once the whole egg has been integrated into the baby's diet, egg yolk alone serves no useful purpose and is thus eliminated from the baby's menu.

Yogurt

When the baby is eating a wide variety of food (cereals, vegetables, fruit, meat, and meat substitutes), yogurt can be added. Ideally, plain yogurt is offered first, either homemade or commercially prepared, without the addition of sugar or fruit. (Homemade yogurt is less sour than the commercial preparation and more easily accepted!)

When a baby is familiar with the flavor of plain yogurt and his appetite is increasing, pieces of mashed fruit can be added (ripe bananas, unsweetened apple sauce, poached pears, etc.).

In the spring of 1979, yogurt in baby-food jars became available. These are undeniably less sweet than ordinary fruit yogurts but do not offer all the benefits of the lactic culture since they are sterilized.

Honey: not before one year!

Since 1975, more than 100 cases of infantile botulism have been reported in the United States and botulism has been accounted for several unexpected baby deaths. Analysis of hundreds of foods either likely, or in fact, actually consumed by the babies, revealed that only honey contained botulism spores and that these spores could cause sudden death in very young children.

These observations have encouraged the Association of Honey Producers of Sioux, Iowa to draw to the public's attention the fact that honey should not be used in baby foods prepared for and ingested by infants under one year of age. Beyond one year, the body can fight the action of the spores if present. Honey should, therefore, not be eaten by babies before twelve months of age.

Fruit Juices

When fruit is introduced, fruit juices can be started as well. Apple juice is the best first choice since it does not cause any allergic reactions. Orange juice can be given next.

Fruit juices are served at room temperature. They are never boiled as heating destroys the vitamin C content, and are served in a small tumbler with a drinking spout rather than in a bottle. Two ounces of juice suffice in meeting vitamin C requirements.

Fruit-flavor crystals, sold in package form, do not contain one iota of fruit and should be avoided even if vitamin C is added.

Processed Meats

Bacon, salted and pressed meats, pâtés and smoked sausages, contain a large amount of salt and fat; they are foods not recommended in a baby's diet, particularly during the first twelve months.

Food mashed with a fork

About six months of age, a baby is better able to chew and easily accepts more consistent food. Food which has been blended is very often replaced by food which is mashed with a fork. From nine to eighteen months of age (see Chapter Twelve), the child usually goes through a transition period during which his diet changes to one which closely resembles that of the family diet, both in variety and texture, with only a few notable exceptions.

Teething Foods

During the long teething period which lasts between four and twenty-four months, certain foods seem to soothe the baby and help him bite and relieve his tender gums. Melba toast and rusks can be useful. However, raw vegetables such as carrots and celery sticks should not be given until the baby is twelve months old. If they are swallowed whole or only partially chewed, they could choke the child.

Pudding custards, cakes, sweet cookies, candies, chocolates, and other such desserts should not be part of the
baby's diet. These "treats" add calories, develop a baby's
sweet tooth, and will lower the nutritive value of the diet
by interfering with a baby's appetite and by replacing more
important foods.

The "Up-To-Date" Report on Commercial Baby Food

A favorite "target" of nutritionists and well-informed
consumers, commercial baby food has turned over a new
leaf in Canada and the United States.

In 1977, the two major Canadian producers of baby
foods eliminated the use of salt in all baby food and reduced
the amount of sugar in all fruit and dessert baby foods.

At least nine types of fruit in jars are currently available
in supermarkets which do not have one gram of sugar
added. For example: apple sauce for babies and juniors,
pear puree for babies and juniors; raisin-and-apple puree
for babies and juniors, prune puree for babies and juniors,
and pineapple-and-pear puree for juniors.

The baby-food industry has to be commended in view of
these vast improvements which encourage good nutritional habits for babies. Some general information about
the content of these baby food jars remains to be added.

Starch content in baby food

Commercial baby food contains a certain amount of either
tapioca, corn starch, barley, or rice flour for proper consistency and to prevent separation of ingredients. These
starches do not affect in any way the nutritional value of
these products, and are not challenged by nutritional
experts, as long as quantities are limited.

Other starches, such as rice and noodles, are part of
"vegetable and meat preparations." These meals compare

favorably with homemade recipes and should not be down-graded if well assimilated into a diet.

Few food additives in these jars

Commercial baby food contains no artificial food colors or flavors. No preservatives are required since these preparations are heated and hermetically sealed in their jars.

Other ingredients in commercial baby food

In order to fully understand baby food labels, a brief explanation about certain terms would be useful.

Reduced iron or electrolytic iron:
- All baby cereals are now enriched with "reduced" iron, also called "electrolytic" iron. These iron particles are more easily absorbed by a baby's digestive system than the other type of iron previously used. For this reason, and because the iron content of regular whole-grain cereals destined for the general population is lower, baby cereals are, by far, the best choice for babies.

Dicalcium phosphate:
- For several years now, manufacturers have been adding calcium and phosphorous, in the form of "dicalcium phosphate," to baby cereals in order to ensure the proper development of bones and teeth, thus complementing the role of milk. This type of enrichment is currently the object of considerable debate.

Citric acid:
- An acid found in fruit which reduces heating time and prevents oxidation in many baby food desserts and fruit purees.

Ascorbic acid:
- A natural emulsifying agent which has been added to a number of cereals in Canada since 1974 and which facilitates the manufacturing process and improves the texture.

Hydrogenated vegetable oil:
- An oil which is added to some baby cereals and desserts in order to improve the texture and the taste.

Bacterial culture:
- A lactic bacteria culture is essential in the manufacture of all yogurts. It is found in baby-food yogurts, but because they are sterilized, the action of these cultures is greatly reduced.

The presence of these food additives is controlled and limited by the Canadian and the American Food and Drug Acts.

Nutritive contents of baby food jars

When a table of food composition for commercial baby foods is consulted, it is evident that the quantity of protein, vitamins, and minerals compares favorably with that of the original food used. Well-chosen commercial baby food is nutritious.

During the first few months during which a baby requires smooth food purees, a mother can choose:
- "plain" vegetables and not creamed or with butter added
- fruit or fruit mixtures, not desserts, custards, or fruit "supremes"
- when meat is first introduced, pureed meats are given; later, "dinners" may be given
- vegetable and meat dinners can occasionally be served at night, when a lighter meal is preferred.

Baby food costs

If a cost comparison is made using the purchasing cost of the foods, commercial baby foods cost twice as much as homemade purees. This difference, which has been verified more than once, applies equally to fruit, vegetables, and meat. The calculation is based on the average cost for a variety of fruit and vegetables, fresh or frozen, as well as meats, poultry, and fish which could be used in preparing homemade purees.

The cost of a blender or a food processor may seem expensive initially, but when the cost is spread over several years of use, it is quite minimal! Who can do without one?

Preparation time is a factor to be considered, but how many mothers calculate the amount of time spent in preparing food? Preparing baby foods can also be done at the same time as other food preparations, and passes almost unnoticed when calculated as part of the total time spent in the kitchen.

CHAPTER TEN

Homemade Baby Food — A New Challenge

A SURVEY CONDUCTED in the Montreal area in November, 1978 showed that one of five mothers served only homemade baby food to her child, while 60% of all mothers surveyed regularly prepared some of their own baby foods while supplementing their babies' diets with commercial baby foods.

Vegetables and fruits are the foods which are most often pureed, followed by poultry, meat, liver, and fish. The baby's diet should be varied and the foods well prepared; however, there are a few cases where the food is too highly salted and sweetened. In Pittsburg, a few years ago, homemade baby foods were analyzed and were often found to contain more salt than commercial baby foods.

If homemade baby food is to contain all of the ingredients essential to health we must be careful not to repeat the past errors of the baby-food producers. It is especially important to watch:

Salt content

1. use only fresh vegetables or salt-free frozen vegetables
2. never use canned vegetable liquid
3. never add salt to baby food either during or after cooking

Sugar content

1. preferably use fresh fruit or unsweetened canned or frozen fruit

2. always discard the sweetened juice from canned fruit and rinse the fruit carefully before placing in the blender
3. avoid the use of sugar, honey, or corn syrup in fruit purees

The Advantages of Homemade Baby Food

As seen in the previous chapter, commercial baby food has significant nutritive value. The systematic elimination of salt and the gradual reduction of sugar from these baby foods has made them quite acceptable from a nutritional standpoint, but one can save a considerable amount of money by preparing homemade baby food. On the basis of the purchasing cost of ingredients only, homemade baby food costs 50% less than commercially prepared foods.

When flavor and variety are considered, homemade baby foods permit the use of a wide variety of vegetables and fish, and allow the use of seasonal foods which are always tasty and full of vitamins.

If nutritive value is considered, homemade baby food, carefully prepared and adequately refrigerated or frozen, retains a large percentage of the original nutrients found in natural food. Homemade preparations are apparently more concentrated since starch is not added. Therefore, portion sizes should be smaller.

An Easy Challenge!

The decision to prepare one's own baby food often reflects a liking for cooking in general as well as a personal conviction that it is the best for the baby.

The suggested method of preparation requires a minimum of time and culinary techniques. It is suggested that small amounts of foods be regularly frozen in individual portions to allow the accumulation of small reserves of food and thereby eliminate last-minute preparations.

The purchase of a blender or a food processor is not essential but they make the task easier. In fact, as the baby needs finely pureed foods for only a limited time, a food mill can also be used.

The Rules of the Game

In order to compete with the hygienic and nutritional qualities of commercially prepared baby food, certain general guidelines should be observed. These may seem exhaustive at first glance but careful reading is needed before going on to the recipe stage.

1. Choose high-quality ingredients

The final quality of pureed foods greatly depends on the quality of the ingredients initially chosen. This, of course, applies to all food preparations but is especially important in the preparation of baby food.

"Fresh" fruit and vegetables that are ripe, and are the proper color and firmness, will always be the best choice. Fruit canned in heavy "sweet" syrup and canned vegetables with a lot of salt are not recommended for baby-food purees. When fresh fruit and vegetables are not available, or are too expensive, unsweetened and unsalted frozen fruit and vegetables with no sauce or flavoring, or fruit canned in its own juice, are suitable alternatives.

Meat, poultry, and fish must also be chosen according to strict rules regarding freshness and quality. Frozen fish is a valid choice, but canned fish generally contains too much salt for a baby under twelve months of age.

2. Vary the menu

A baby eating a consistent diet of carrots and potatoes, six or seven days a week, is not eating a varied diet! The essential nutrients favorable to growth and health are only found in a variety of food. New foods and new flavors are easily accepted by a baby, and since this is a period of large appetites and of few food whims, you must take advantage of this!

You can alternate green and yellow vegetables on the

menu and gradually add potatoes as the baby's appetite increases. Either lean meat, poultry, or fish should be selected to provide variety at the main daily meal. The need to offer a variety of food to the baby does not mean an increase in the preparation time at each meal. Thanks to the freezer, you can prepare food when you feel like it, or when time permits, and freeze it in individual portions for future meals.

3. Follow a few hygienic rules

In order to eliminate the possibility of food contamination and to protect the baby from infections, certain simple rules should be observed:
- wash hands well before handling any food which will be used to prepare homemade baby food
- use utensils and containers that have been impeccably cleaned
- cover the food well once cooked and refrigerate immediately; do not let sit at room temperature
- when baby food is prepared in small quantities and unfrozen, do not keep the food more than three days in the refrigerator
- do not refreeze a thawed puree.

4. Assemble the necessary utensils

Since solids or homemade purees are introduced only between four and six months of age, very smooth purees or purees without lumps need only be prepared for a few months. From six to eight months, a baby's chewing ability enables him to easily eat food mashed by a fork. A blender or food processor will make the job much easier. However, if you do not wish to invest in such expensive appliances, an inexpensive manual food mill can also be used.

The following utensils will also be needed: containers, measuring cups and measuring spoons, individual ice-cube containers, freezer bags with ties (capacity: 1 pint, or 1 quart, depending on the quantities to be prepared), small aluminum plates, labels.

5. Cook the food rapidly

Cooking makes digestion easier. In addition, when done properly, it retains the highest percentage of nutrients. Vegetables should be either steamed or cooked in a small amount of boiling water in order to minimize vitamin losses. Rapid-cooking periods are preferable to prolonged cooking periods. Tender yet firm vegetables contain more vitamins than limp and discolored vegetables. Obviously, frozen vegetables should not be thawed before cooking, and the cooking period must be very short.

It is recommended that poultry, meat, or fish be cooked in a certain amount of liquid. Fresh fruit, on the other hand, is peeled and poached in a small amount of un-sweetened water or fruit juice, except for ripe bananas which can simply be mashed with a fork or pureed in the blender.

Cooking water should be used as much as possible in preparing purees because quite a few of the nutrients present in vegetables, meat, or fruit remain in the water after cooking.

6. Puree rapidly

Cooked food which has been cooled slightly is placed into the blender. The consistency of the puree will vary depending on a baby's age, but overblending should be avoided in order to minimize the loss of nutrients. For a more liquid puree, more cooking water is added and the mixture is blended again. As a general rule, if the food takes too long to liquify, the amount of liquid may be insufficient or the pieces of food could be too large or too numerous. One and one-half to two cups of food can be pureed at one time. However, in the cases of poultry or meat, only one cup (250 mL) should be used. Additional quantities hamper the operation of the blender and the final quality of the product is affected.

7. Pour into containers and cool

Once the puree is finished, it is poured into ice-cube containers. Each cube contains about two ounces of food.

The puree is then cooled in the refrigerator before freezing.

8. Freeze

The cooled ice-cube containers are then covered with a sheet of waxed paper and placed in the coldest part of the freezer, far from the door. Eight to twelve hours are needed for freezing to take place. Purees can be kept in the freezer for varying lengths of time, depending on the ingredients. The following table shows the maximum time for which various homemade purees may be kept frozen at 0°F (-18°C).

X-1: *Freezer Storage Time for Homemade Purees*

Food	Freezing Period
vegetables	6 to 8 months
fruits	6 to 8 months
fruits with tapioca	6 weeks
meat and poultry, cooked (chicken, veal, beef, turkey)	10 weeks
fish, cooked	10 weeks
vegetable and meat meal	10 weeks
purees containing milk	4 to 6 weeks

9. Place frozen purees in plastic bags

Once the purees are frozen, remove the ice-cube trays from the freezer and empty the individually frozen purees into small polyethylene bags, one type of food per bag. The bag is then sealed after withdrawing the air with a straw, and is properly labelled as to the type of food as well as the preparation date. The bags are then returned to the freezer.

10. Take out one or two cubes from the bag and warm in a double boiler

At mealtime, the desired number of cubes is removed from the freezer bags. Vegetables, meat, and poultry are then warmed in a double boiler. Fruit requires less thawing time.

NOTE: If last-minute preparation involving a small quantity of food is desired, steps one to six are followed. The puree stored in a closed container can be kept in the refrigerator three days without any problems.

It is strongly recommended that vegetables, fruit and meat be given plain at the start. Once the baby has tasted the individual flavors, mixtures, such as apples and pears, can be offered.

11. Heating baby foods in the microwave

Many homemade as well as commercial foods may be heated in the microwave oven. Here are some important tips to follow:

— Baby foods that contain substantial amounts of meat should not be heated in microwave ovens. Plain meats, poultry, high meat dinners, egg yolks and meat sticks should be warmed by conventional methods. Microwave heating of these foods results in uneven heating that could cause the jar to explode. Droplets of water in the food heat faster by microwaves than the dense protein and fat particles. The water turns to steam in small pockets. Shaking the jar or dish when removing from the microwave or just stirring the food with a spoon could lead to a hot splatter or scald.

— To heat a food item, put it either in a dish or, if in a baby jar, place the *opened* jar on a plate, and insert into the oven. Be sure to remove any caps and leave them outside the oven. Start the oven on the warm setting, or at the lowest level of heat, and test frequently until the food reaches feeding temperature. You may want to record the time and temperature for future reference. Avoid overheating.

— Consult the manufacturer's instruction booklet or your dealer before putting baby food in the microwave.

— Reusable baby bottles containing milk may be warmed in the microwave; observe the same precautions as with baby foods listed above. Overheating causes milk to boil over the bottle rim. Bottles should not have the caps or nipples on when being warmed. Disposable baby bottles (bags) should not be microwave heated.

RECIPES

Puree of Carrots

Ingredients
2 lb. (1 kg) fresh carrots
Water
Preparation
1. Peel carrots and cut into 1 inch (2.5 cm) pieces. Place them into a small amount of boiling water. Cover and simmer 20 to 30 minutes or until tender.
2. Place 1½ cups (375 mL) of the carrots and ⅓ cup (85 mL) of fresh water into the blender. Puree. Repeat with the remaining carrots. Pour into ice-cube trays and freeze.

Yield
2 ice-cube trays
Storage Life
6 to 8 months
Comments
Fresh carrots are always a better buy than the frozen or canned variety; they can be cooked in a pressure cooker or steamed before they are pureed. Carrots represent an excellent choice because babies are usually fond of them and they also provide an excellent source of vitamin A.

NOTE: Despite certain warnings about the use of homemade carrot purees, this vegetable does not present any problems if carefully prepared with fresh water, refrigerated, and then frozen rapidly, especially when it is offered to a baby who is older than four months.

Puree of Green Bean

Ingredients
1½ lb. (700 g) fresh and tender green beans
1 teaspoon (5 g) minced onion (optional)
Water
Preparation
1. Wash the beans; top and tail them and cut into thirds. Place beans and onions into a small amount of boiling water. Cover and simmer for 20 to 25 minutes or until beans are tender but still bright green. Remove from heat and cool slightly.
2. Place half of the cooked beans and ⅓ cup (85 mL) of the cooking water into

the blender. Puree. Repeat
with remaining beans.
3. Pour into ice-cube trays
and freeze.
Yield
2 ice-cube trays
Storage life
6 to 8 months
Comments
To make good puree, green
beans must be young and
tender. Frozen green beans
may also be used in this
recipe.
NOTE: Start with plain
beans without the onion at
first, then proceed to a
combination of flavors later
on.

Puree of Sweet Potato

1½ lb. (700 g) sweet potato
(2 medium potatoes)
Water
Preparation
1. Peel and cut potatoes into
slices about ¾" (2 cm)
thick. Place in 1½ cups
(375 mL) of boiling water;
simmer for 30 to 45
minutes or until potatoes
are tender. Remove from
heat and cool slightly.
2. Place 1 cup (250 mL) of
the cooked potatoes and ½
cup (125 mL) of the
cooking water into the
blender. Puree. Repeat
with the remaining
vegetable. Pour into ice-
cube trays and freeze.

Yield
2 ice-cube trays
Storage Life
6 months
Comments
Sweet potatoes are the candy
of vegetables and contain a
lot of vitamin A.

Puree of Beet

1 lb. (500 g) beets
(approximately 6 small beets)
Water
Preparation
1. Wash beets, cut stalks off
2" (95 cm) from the top of
the vegetable; do not peel
beets.
2. Place unpeeled beets into 1
cup (250 mL) of boiling
water. Simmer for 30 to
60 minutes or until beets
are tender (age and size of
beets affect cooking time).
Remove from heat and
cool slightly.
3. Peel and slice cooked
beets. Place into the
blender. Add ¼ to ⅓ cup
(60 to 85 mL) of fresh
water, not the cooking
water. Puree. Pour into
ice-cube trays and freeze.
Yield
1 ice-cube tray
Storage Life
6 months
Comments
Whole beets can also be
cooked in the pressure cooker
or steamed before they are

pureed; well-drained canned beets may also be used. When beets are served, a bib for both mother and baby is a good idea. Serve this vegetable after six months of age and only occasionally.

Mixed Vegetable Puree

Ingredients
2 cups (500 mL) mixed vegetables (4 carrots, 4 parsnips, sliced)
2 cups (500 mL) peeled and sliced potatoes (2 average potatoes)
Water
Preparation
1. Peel and cut the vegetables into pieces; place all vegetables, except the potatoes, into 1 cup (250 mL) of boiling water. Simmer for 10 minutes. Add the potatoes and simmer until all vegetables are tender (about 20 minutes). Remove from heat and cool slightly.
2. Place into the blender 1 cup (250 mL) of the cooked vegetables and about ⅓ cup (85 mL) of the cooking water. Puree. Repeat with the remaining vegetables. Pour into ice-cube trays and freeze.
Yield
2 ice-cube trays
Storage Life
6 months

Comments
Carrots and parsnips can be replaced by turnip, rutabaga, or another root vegetable.
NOTE: This puree should be served only after each individual vegetable has been introduced to the baby first.

Puree of Squash

Ingredients
1 squash
Water
Preparation
1. Bake the whole squash in a 350°F (180°C) oven for about 1½ hours. Once cooked, cut in half and remove seeds and skin.
2. Place the fleshy part of the squash and a small amount of water (¼ cup/ 60 mL or more) into the blender. Puree. Pour into ice-cube trays and freeze.
Yield
1 ice-cube tray or more, depending on the size of the squash
Storage Life
6 months
Comments
Frozen squash can be used in this recipe. The whole squash family supplies good quantities of vitamin A.

Squash and Apple Puree

Ingredients
1½ cups (375 mL) fresh squash cut into pieces

3 to 4 apples, peeled and sliced

Water

Preparation

1. Place apples and pieces of squash into 1 cup (250 mL) of boiling water. Simmer for 25 to 30 minutes or until apples and squash are tender. Remove from heat and cool slightly.

2. Place one-half of the apple-squash mixture into the blender along with ⅓ cup (85 mL) of the cooking water. Puree. Repeat with the remaining ingredients. Pour into ice-cube trays and freeze.

Yield

2 ice-cube trays

Storage Life

6 months

Comments

A pleasant way to eat squash, a vegetable which provides an excellent source of vitamin A.

Puree of Zucchini

Ingredients

1½ lb. (700 g) young zucchini (7 to 8 small ones)

Water

Preparation

1. Peel and slice zucchinis. Place into 1 cup of boiling water or into a steamer. Simmer gently for about 15 minutes. Remove from heat, drain well, and cool slightly.

2. Place into the blender without any water. Puree. Repeat with the remaining cooked zucchini.

3. Pour into ice-cube trays and freeze.

Yield

2 ice-cube trays

Storage Life

6 months

Comments

Zucchini is sweet and pleasant tasting. The puree appears as a pretty "spring green."

Puree of Asparagus

Ingredients

1 lb. (500 g) tender and young asparagus (in season)

Water

1 tablespoon of sweet butter or margarine

Preparation

1. Wash and cut asparagus into 2" (95 cm) pieces. Place into about ½ cup (125 mL) of boiling water. Simmer for 10 to 15 minutes or until the asparagus is tender. Remove from heat and cool slightly.

2. Place into the blender half of the asparagus and a small amount of cooking water. Puree. Repeat with the remaining asparagus. Add butter or margarine

to the puree. Pour into
ice-cube trays and freeze.
Yield
1 ice-cube tray
Storage Life
6 months
Comments
A real spring delicacy.

Puree of Cauliflower

Ingredients
1 small head of cauliflower
Water
½ cup (125 mL) of whole
milk*
Preparation
1. Section the cauliflower
   into small flowerettes.
   Place into 1 cup (250 mL)
   of boiling water. Simmer
   for 15 to 20 minutes or
   until the cauliflower is
   tender. Remove from heat
   and cool slightly.
2. Place into the blender with
   1½ cups (375 mL) of the
   cooking water and half the
   milk. Puree. Repeat with
   the remaining ingredients.
   Pour into ice-cube trays
   and freeze.
Yield
2 ice-cube trays, depending
on the size of the cauliflower
Storage Life
4 to 6 weeks
Comments
Cauliflower absorbs a lot of
liquid while cooking; this is
the reason for adding milk
when making the puree.

As with all members of the
cabbage family, cauliflower is
rich in vitamin C.
   *Do not give 2%, 1% or
skim milk to a baby under
one year of age.

Puree of Broccoli

Ingredients
1 bunch of fresh (green)
broccoli (5 to 6 stalks)
Water
Preparation
1. Cut the stalks and retain
   only the flower part of the
   broccoli for baby purees
   (the stalks may be cooked
   and served along with
   another vegetable to the
   rest of the family).
2. Place the pieces of broccoli
   into 1 cup (250 mL) of
   boiling water. Simmer for
   15 minutes or until the
   broccoli is tender but still
   very green. Remove from
   heat and cool slightly.
3. Place half of the broccoli
   along with ¼ cup (60 mL)
   of the cooking water into
   the blender. Puree. Repeat
   with the remaining
   broccoli. Pour into ice-
   cube trays and freeze.
Yield
1 ice-cube tray
Storage Life
6 months
Comments
Fresh and bright green
broccoli has a sweet and

pleasant flavor. It is rich in vitamins A and C. It also contains iron and calcium.

Apple Sauce or Compote

Ingredients
8 to 10 medium apples
Water
Cinnamon (optional)
Preparation
1. Wash apples well. Remove cores, cut into quarters, and slice. Place apples in a saucepan with ½ cup (125 mL) of water. Bring to a boil, reduce heat and simmer for about 20 minutes or until apples are tender.
2. Remove from heat and cool slightly.
3. Place 2 cups (500 mL) of the cooked apples into the blender and puree until the peel has completely disappeared. (If the blender is not powerful enough to pulverize the peel entirely, pass the puree through a sieve or peel apples before cooking.)
4. Repeat with the remaining apples.
5. If desired, a pinch of cinnamon may be added to the puree.
6. Pour into ice cube trays and freeze.
Yield
2 ice-cube trays

Storage Life
6 to 8 months
Comments
Cooking time may vary according to the type of apple used.

Puree of Pear

Ingredients
9 to 11 medium pears (fresh)
½ cup (125 mL) water or apple juice
Preparation
1. Peel pears, quarter and core.
2. Place into a saucepan with ½ cup (125 mL) of water or apple juice. Simmer for 20 to 30 minutes or until pears are tender. Remove from heat and cool slightly.
3. Place half of the cooked pears into the blender with ⅛ cup (20 mL) of the cooking liquid. Puree. Repeat with the remaining pears.
4. Pour puree into ice-cube trays and freeze.
Yield
2 ice-cube trays
Storage Life
6 to 8 months
Comments
If canned pears are used, they should be carefully rinsed to eliminate as much sugar as possible; they should not be cooked. However, unsweetened pears canned in

their natural juice are now available; this juice may be used as the liquid in the making of the puree.

Puree of Pear and Apple

Ingredients
5 apples and 5 pears
½ cup (125 mL) water or apple juice, approximately

Preparation
1. Peel apples and pears; quarter and core them.
2. Place into a saucepan with the water or the apple juice and simmer for 20 to 25 minutes or until the apples and pears are tender.
3. Remove from heat and cool slightly.
4. Place half the fruit into the blender with about ¼ cup (60 mL) of the cooking liquid. Puree. Repeat with the remaining fruit.
5. Pour into ice-cube trays.

Yield
2 ice-cube trays

Storage Life
6 to 8 months

Comments
The amounts of liquid may vary depending on the type of apples and pears used.

A fruit puree can be made by mashing cooked fruit with a fork.

Puree of Peach

Ingredients
4 cups (1 liter) fresh peaches, peeled, pitted, and sliced
⅓ to ½ cup (85 to 125 mL) water

Preparation
1. Put peaches and water into a saucepan. Bring to a boil, reduce heat and simmer gently for about 15 to 20 minutes or until peaches are tender.
2. Remove from heat and cool slightly.
3. Place 2 cups (500 mL) of cooked peaches into the blender together with a very small amount of the cooking water. Puree.
4. Repeat with the remaining peaches.
5. Pour into ice-cube trays and freeze.

Yield
2 ice-cube trays

Storage Life
6 to 8 months

Comments
Avoid adding too much water when blending. The amount required will depend on the type of peaches used. If canned peaches are used, they must be rinsed well in order to eliminate as much of the sugar as possible. They do not have to be cooked before blending. Peaches canned in grape or un-

sweetened fruit juice are also available on the market. This liquid may be used to replace the cooking water when making the puree.

apricots which have been carefully rinsed may be used but do not cook. Apricots are a good source of vitamin A.

Puree of Apricot

Ingredients
4 cups (1 liter) unpeeled fresh apricots, pitted and sliced
½ cup (125 mL) water, approximately
Preparation
1. Place apricots and water into a saucepan. Bring to a boil, reduce heat. Simmer for about 15 minutes or until fruit is tender.
2. Remove from heat and cool slightly.
3. Place half of the apricots into the blender with about ¼ cup (60 mL) of the cooking water. Puree. Repeat with the remaining apricots.
4. Pour into ice-cube trays and freeze.
Yield
2 ice-cube trays
Storage Life
6 to 8 months
Comments
As with peaches, do not add too much water when blending. One part of the apricots may be replaced with either apples or pears (2 cups (500 mL) pears, 2 cups (500 mL) apricots. Again, canned

Puree of Prune and Apple

Ingredients
1½ cups (375 mL) pitted prunes (350 g or 12-oz. bag)
2 cups (500 mL) hot water
2 cups (500 mL) peeled, sliced, cored apples
1½ cups (375 mL) cold water
Preparation
1. Soak prunes in hot water for 5 to 15 minutes; drain.
2. Place prunes, apples, and cold water into a saucepan; bring to a boil; reduce heat and simmer for about 20 minutes.
3. Remove from heat and cool slightly.
4. Place half of the prunes and apples and about ½ cup (125 mL) of the cooking water into the blender. Puree. Repeat with the remaining fruit.
5. Pour into ice-cube trays.
Yield
2 ice-cube trays
Storage Life
6 months
Comments
This puree could be the solution in the case of an infant who is constipated and does not eliminate regularly.

If the prunes when purchased are not pitted, the pits are easily removed after the 15-minute soak. When mashed with a fork, the fruit resembles a puree.

Puree of Veal

Ingredients
1 lb. (500 g) boneless lean veal, cut in 1½" (4 cm) cubes
3 carrots, peeled and cut into pieces
2 potatoes, peeled and quartered
1 tablespoon (15 g) minced onion
1 stalk of celery, cut into pieces
Water

Preparation
1. Place all ingredients into a saucepan with 2 cups (500 mL) of water. Bring to a boil; reduce heat. Simmer for approximately 45 minutes, or until veal and vegetables are tender. Remove from heat and cool slightly.
2. Separate the cooked veal from the vegetable. Place half the meat and ½ cup (125 mL) of the stock into the blender. Puree. Repeat with remaining veal.
3. Pour into ice-cube trays and freeze.

Yield
12 small cubes

Storage Life
10 to 12 weeks

Comments
The vegetables may also be pureed with or without a small amount of veal to produce a "vegetable and veal" dinner. Veal is very expensive. It adds variety to the baby's diet, but it is not indispensable.

Puree of Beef

Ingredients
1 lb. (500 g) lean, tender beef (top or sirloin) cut into 1" (2.5 cm) cubes
1 stalk of celery cut into pieces
3 carrots, peeled and cut into pieces
2 medium potatoes, peeled and quartered
1 tablespoon (15 g) minced onion
Water

Preparation
1. Place beef and 2¼ cups (560 mL) of water into a saucepan; simmer for about 45 minutes.
2. Add celery, carrots and potatoes and cook for an additional 35 to 40 minutes, or until all ingredients are tender. Remove from heat and cool slightly.
3. Separate the beef from the vegetables and place ¾ cup

(180 mL) of the meat into the blender with ⅓ cup (85 mL) of the stock. Puree. Repeat with remaining beef. Pour into ice-cube trays and freeze.

Yield
12 small cubes
Storage Life
10 to 12 weeks
Comments
The vegetables may be pureed with a small amount of beef to make a "vegetable and beef" dinner.

3. Pour into ice-cube trays and freeze.

Yield
6 cubes
Storage Life
10 to 12 weeks
Comments
Liver is an excellent source of iron and protein. Chicken livers have a milder flavor than other types of livers. With a small amount of sweet potato or another "favorite" vegetable, it's a guaranteed success.

Puree of Chicken Livers

Ingredients
5 to 6 chicken livers
Unsalted chicken stock (homemade)
Preparation
1. Prepare livers for cooking by cutting and removing the white membrane; cut livers in half. Place into a saucepan with 1 cup (250 mL) of unsalted chicken stock. Bring to a boil; reduce heat immediately. Simmer 5 to 10 minutes, or until chicken livers are cooked (grey-brown inside). Remove from heat and cool slightly.
2. Place a few chicken livers into the blender with a small amount of cooking liquid. Puree. Repeat with remaining liver.

Puree of Chicken

Ingredients
1 chicken, 2 to 3 lb. (1 to 1.3 kg) cut into 4 to 8 pieces
1 stalk of celery cut into pieces
1 tablespoon (15 g) minced onion
1 sprig of parsley
3 carrots, peeled and cut into pieces
1 medium potato, peeled and quartered
Preparation
1. Place chicken, celery, onion and parsley into a saucepan. Add 3 cups (750 mL) of water. Simmer for 40 to 50 minutes.
2. Add the vegetables (carrots and potato). Simmer for an additional 40 to 45 minutes or until the chicken is cooked and

the meat separates easily from the bones.

3. Remove from heat and cool slightly.

4. Remove the meat from the bones and cut into small pieces. Place ½ cup (125 mL) of chicken and ⅓ cup (85 mL) of the stock into the blender. Puree. Repeat with remaining chicken.

5. Pour puree into ice-cube trays and freeze.

Yield
One tray of cubes or more, depending on the size of the chicken.

Storage Life
10 to 12 weeks

Comments
Turkey can easily replace chicken in the recipe; frozen turkey halves or quarters can be purchased and cooked in the same manner as the chicken.

NOTE: The vegetables may be pureed with a small amount of chicken to make a "vegetable and chicken" dinner.

Puree of Fish

Ingredients
2 white fish fillets (sole, cod, ocean, perch, haddock) 8 oz.
(200 g) approximately
1 to 2 tablespoons (15 to 30 g) finely minced onion
½ cup (125 mL) whole milk*

Preparation
1. Pour ¼ cup (60 mL) of milk into a frying pan and heat gently. Add the onion; cook for a few minutes.

2. Add the fish filets. Cover with a lid or aluminum foil. Cook over slow heat for 5 to 10 minutes or until the fish is very white and flakes easily with a fork. Remove from heat and cool slightly.

3. Place half of the fish and the milk used in cooking into the blender. Blend until smooth; add more milk if necessary. Repeat with the remaining fish. Pour into ice-cube trays and freeze.

Yield
8 cubes

Storage Life
4 to 6 weeks

Comments
White fish is an excellent source of protein. It contains less fat than meat and its preparation is faster. It has a mild and pleasant flavor.

*Do not give 2%, 1% or skim milk to a baby under one year of age.

CHAPTER ELEVEN

Some Very Special Flowers Talk About Nutrition

TRANSLATING VITAMINS and minerals into daily nutritional needs is not that complicated. In order to ease the process and to better understand the different nutritional needs of the young child, this chapter presents a summary of fourteen essential nutrients.

Each flower represents a specific nutrient and the parts of each flower reveal pertinent nutritional information. The heart of the flower represents its role, while the petals indicate the major food sources of the nutrient. The leaves represent the child's daily needs both in technical terms and in terms of actual food portions. How cooking affects the nutrient completes the information.

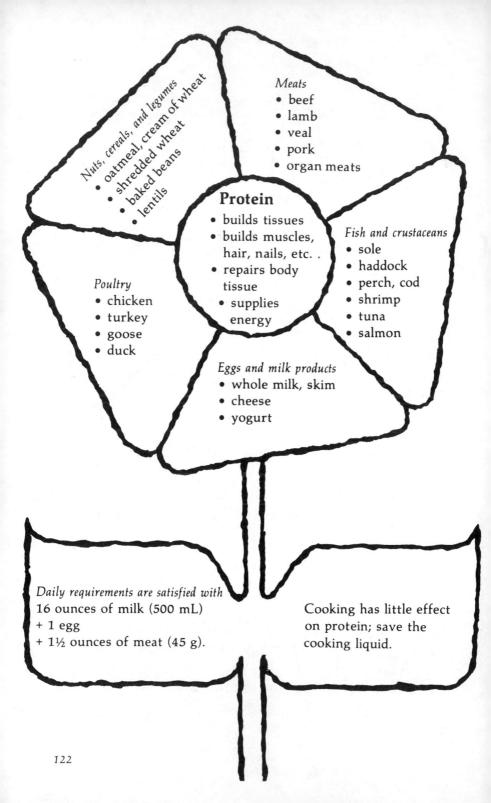

Nuts, cereals, and legumes
- oatmeal, cream of wheat
- shredded wheat
- baked beans
- lentils

Meats
- beef
- lamb
- veal
- pork
- organ meats

Protein
- builds tissues
- builds muscles, hair, nails, etc. .
- repairs body tissue
- supplies energy

Fish and crustaceans
- sole
- haddock
- perch, cod
- shrimp
- tuna
- salmon

Poultry
- chicken
- turkey
- goose
- duck

Eggs and milk products
- whole milk, skim
- cheese
- yogurt

Daily requirements are satisfied with
16 ounces of milk (500 mL)
+ 1 egg
+ 1½ ounces of meat (45 g).

Cooking has little effect on protein; save the cooking liquid.

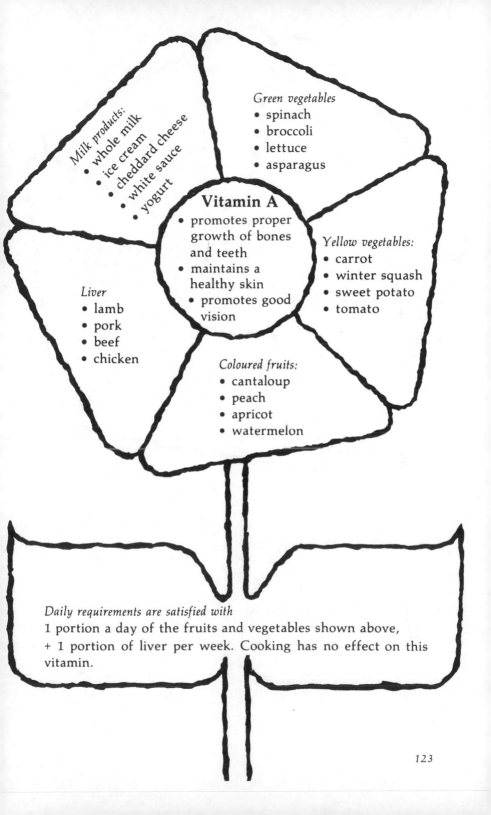

Milk products:
- whole milk
- ice cream
- cheddard cheese
- white sauce
- yogurt

Green vegetables
- spinach
- broccoli
- lettuce
- asparagus

Vitamin A
- promotes proper growth of bones and teeth
- maintains a healthy skin
- promotes good vision

Yellow vegetables:
- carrot
- winter squash
- sweet potato
- tomato

Liver
- lamb
- pork
- beef
- chicken

Coloured fruits:
- cantaloup
- peach
- apricot
- watermelon

Daily requirements are satisfied with
1 portion a day of the fruits and vegetables shown above,
+ 1 portion of liver per week. Cooking has no effect on this vitamin.

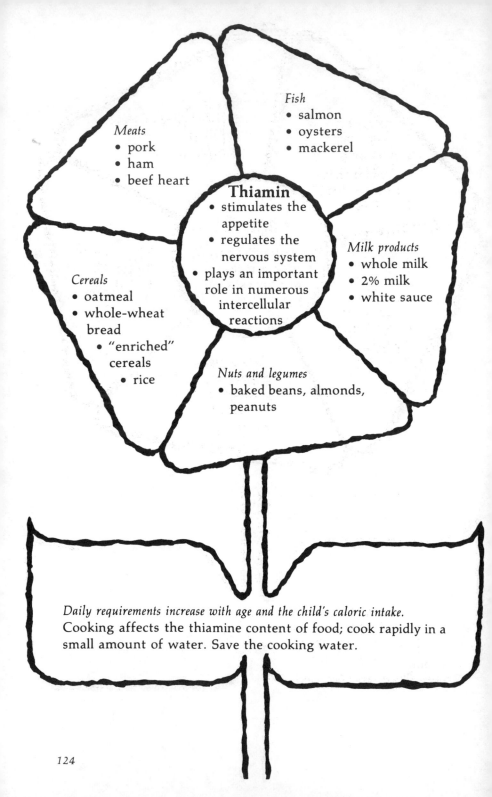

Thiamin
- stimulates the appetite
- regulates the nervous system
- plays an important role in numerous intercellular reactions

Meats
- pork
- ham
- beef heart

Fish
- salmon
- oysters
- mackerel

Milk products
- whole milk
- 2% milk
- white sauce

Nuts and legumes
- baked beans, almonds, peanuts

Cereals
- oatmeal
- whole-wheat bread
- "enriched" cereals
- rice

Daily requirements increase with age and the child's caloric intake. Cooking affects the thiamine content of food; cook rapidly in a small amount of water. Save the cooking water.

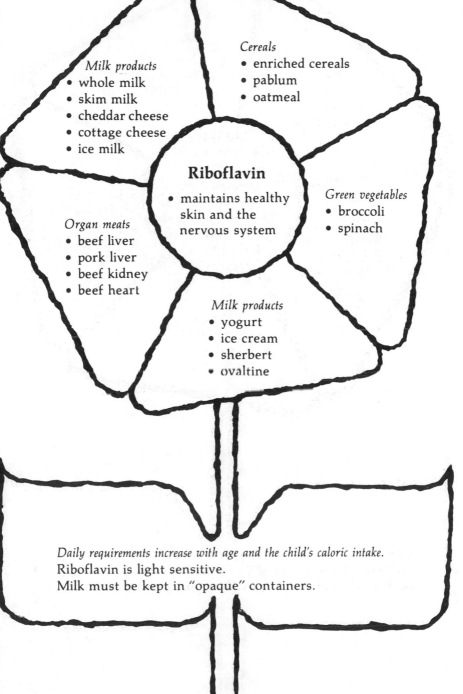

Milk products
- whole milk
- skim milk
- cheddar cheese
- cottage cheese
- ice milk

Cereals
- enriched cereals
- pablum
- oatmeal

Riboflavin
- maintains healthy skin and the nervous system

Green vegetables
- broccoli
- spinach

Organ meats
- beef liver
- pork liver
- beef kidney
- beef heart

Milk products
- yogurt
- ice cream
- sherbert
- ovaltine

Daily requirements increase with age and the child's caloric intake.
Riboflavin is light sensitive.
Milk must be kept in "opaque" containers.

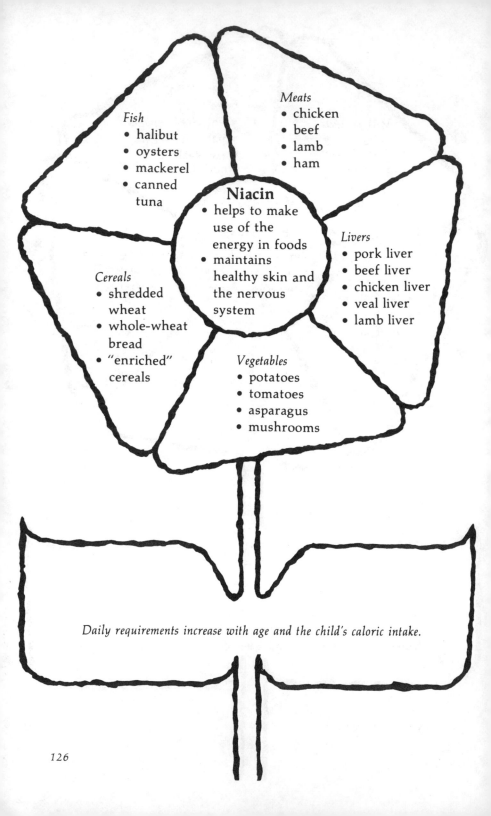

Niacin
- helps to make use of the energy in foods
- maintains healthy skin and the nervous system

Fish
- halibut
- oysters
- mackerel
- canned tuna

Meats
- chicken
- beef
- lamb
- ham

Livers
- pork liver
- beef liver
- chicken liver
- veal liver
- lamb liver

Cereals
- shredded wheat
- whole-wheat bread
- "enriched" cereals

Vegetables
- potatoes
- tomatoes
- asparagus
- mushrooms

Daily requirements increase with age and the child's caloric intake.

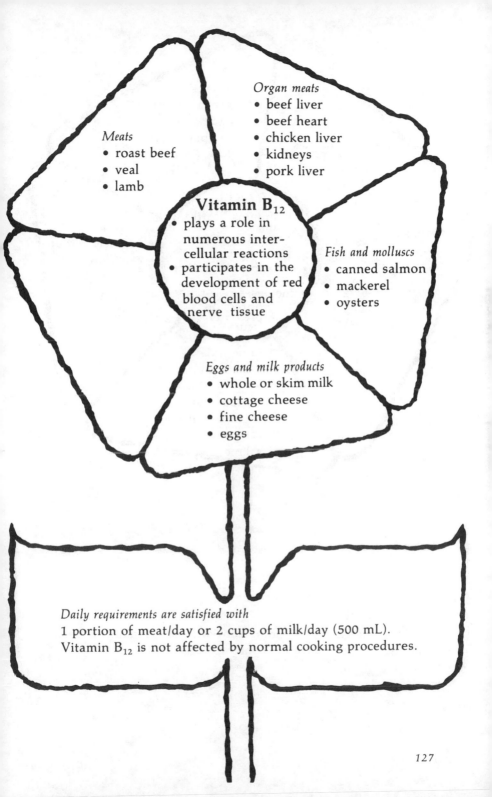

Meats
• roast beef
• veal
• lamb

Organ meats
• beef liver
• beef heart
• chicken liver
• kidneys
• pork liver

Vitamin B$_{12}$
• plays a role in numerous inter-cellular reactions
• participates in the development of red blood cells and nerve tissue

Fish and molluscs
• canned salmon
• mackerel
• oysters

Eggs and milk products
• whole or skim milk
• cottage cheese
• fine cheese
• eggs

Daily requirements are satisfied with
1 portion of meat/day or 2 cups of milk/day (500 mL).
Vitamin B$_{12}$ is not affected by normal cooking procedures.

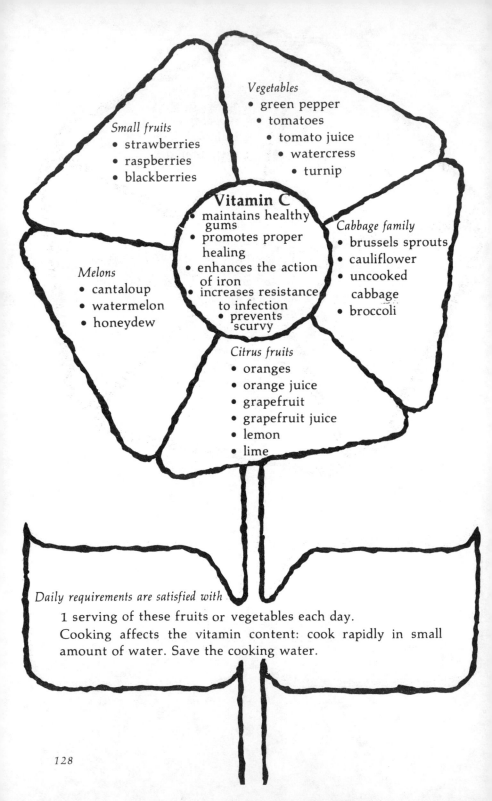

Vitamin C
- maintains healthy gums
- promotes proper healing
- enhances the action of iron
- increases resistance to infection
- prevents scurvy

Small fruits
- strawberries
- raspberries
- blackberries

Vegetables
- green pepper
- tomatoes
- tomato juice
- watercress
- turnip

Cabbage family
- brussels sprouts
- cauliflower
- uncooked cabbage
- broccoli

Melons
- cantaloup
- watermelon
- honeydew

Citrus fruits
- oranges
- orange juice
- grapefruit
- grapefruit juice
- lemon
- lime

Daily requirements are satisfied with
1 serving of these fruits or vegetables each day.
Cooking affects the vitamin content: cook rapidly in small amount of water. Save the cooking water.

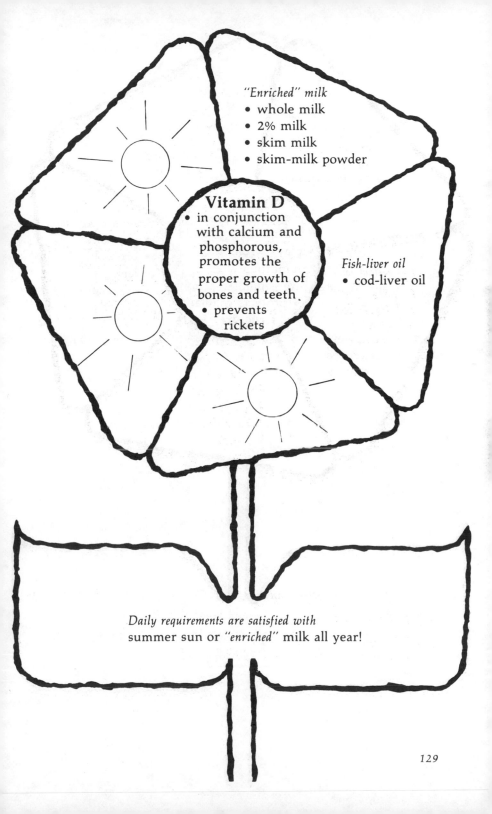

"Enriched" milk
• whole milk
• 2% milk
• skim milk
• skim-milk powder

Vitamin D
• in conjunction with calcium and phosphorous, promotes the proper growth of bones and teeth
• prevents rickets

Fish-liver oil
• cod-liver oil

Daily requirements are satisfied with summer sun or *"enriched"* milk all year!

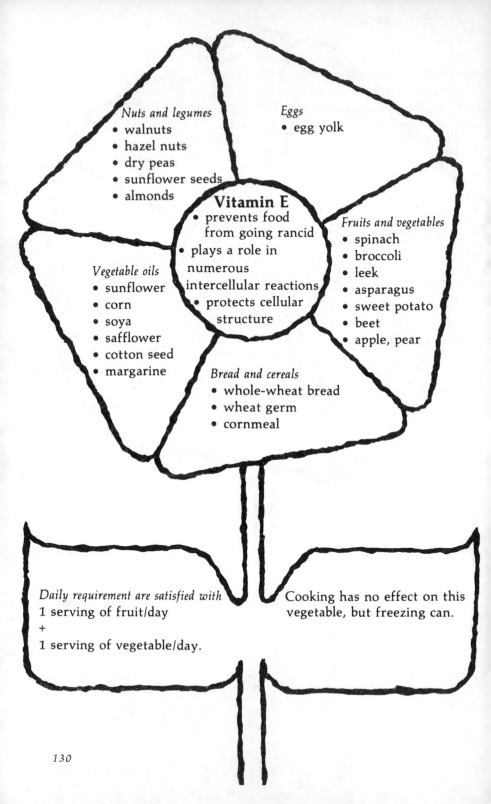

Vitamin E
- prevents food from going rancid
- plays a role in numerous intercellular reactions
- protects cellular structure

Nuts and legumes
- walnuts
- hazel nuts
- dry peas
- sunflower seeds
- almonds

Eggs
- egg yolk

Fruits and vegetables
- spinach
- broccoli
- leek
- asparagus
- sweet potato
- beet
- apple, pear

Vegetable oils
- sunflower
- corn
- soya
- safflower
- cotton seed
- margarine

Bread and cereals
- whole-wheat bread
- wheat germ
- cornmeal

Daily requirement are satisfied with 1 serving of fruit/day
+
1 serving of vegetable/day.

Cooking has no effect on this vegetable, but freezing can.

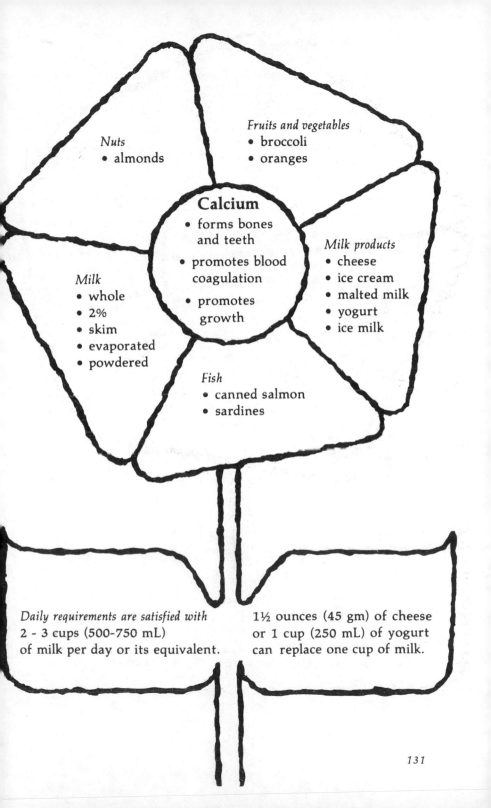

Nuts
• almonds

Fruits and vegetables
• broccoli
• oranges

Calcium
• forms bones and teeth
• promotes blood coagulation
• promotes growth

Milk products
• cheese
• ice cream
• malted milk
• yogurt
• ice milk

Milk
• whole
• 2%
• skim
• evaporated
• powdered

Fish
• canned salmon
• sardines

Daily requirements are satisfied with 2 - 3 cups (500-750 mL) of milk per day or its equivalent.

1½ ounces (45 gm) of cheese or 1 cup (250 mL) of yogurt can replace one cup of milk.

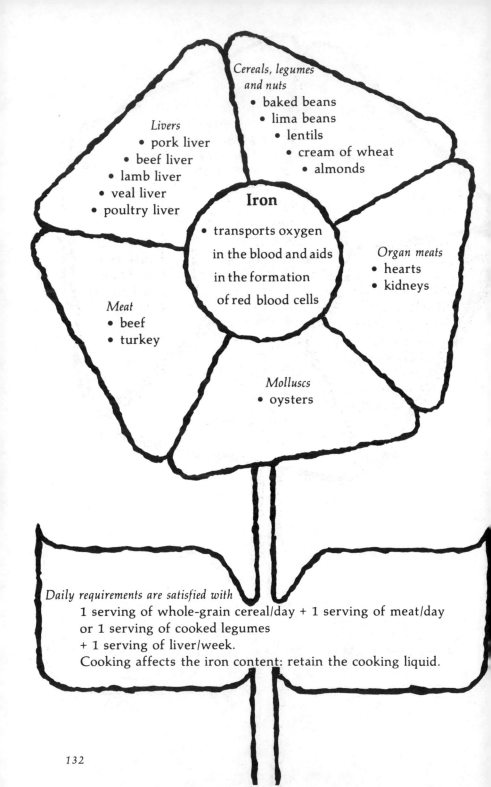

Iron

• transports oxygen
in the blood and aids
in the formation
of red blood cells

Livers
• pork liver
• beef liver
• lamb liver
• veal liver
• poultry liver

*Cereals, legumes
and nuts*
• baked beans
• lima beans
• lentils
• cream of wheat
• almonds

Organ meats
• hearts
• kidneys

Meat
• beef
• turkey

Molluscs
• oysters

Daily requirements are satisfied with
1 serving of whole-grain cereal/day + 1 serving of meat/day
or 1 serving of cooked legumes
+ 1 serving of liver/week.
Cooking affects the iron content: retain the cooking liquid.

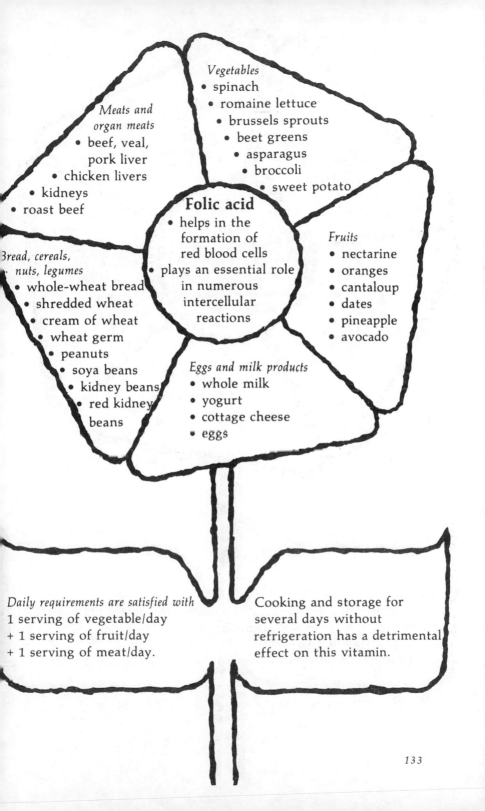

Vegetables
- spinach
- romaine lettuce
- brussels sprouts
- beet greens
- asparagus
- broccoli
- sweet potato

Meats and
organ meats
- beef, veal,
pork liver
- chicken livers
- kidneys
- roast beef

Folic acid
- helps in the
formation of
red blood cells
- plays an essential role
in numerous
intercellular
reactions

Fruits
- nectarine
- oranges
- cantaloup
- dates
- pineapple
- avocado

Bread, cereals,
nuts, legumes
- whole-wheat bread
- shredded wheat
- cream of wheat
- wheat germ
- peanuts
- soya beans
- kidney beans
- red kidney
beans

Eggs and milk products
- whole milk
- yogurt
- cottage cheese
- eggs

Daily requirements are satisfied with
1 serving of vegetable/day
+ 1 serving of fruit/day
+ 1 serving of meat/day.

Cooking and storage for
several days without
refrigeration has a detrimental
effect on this vitamin.

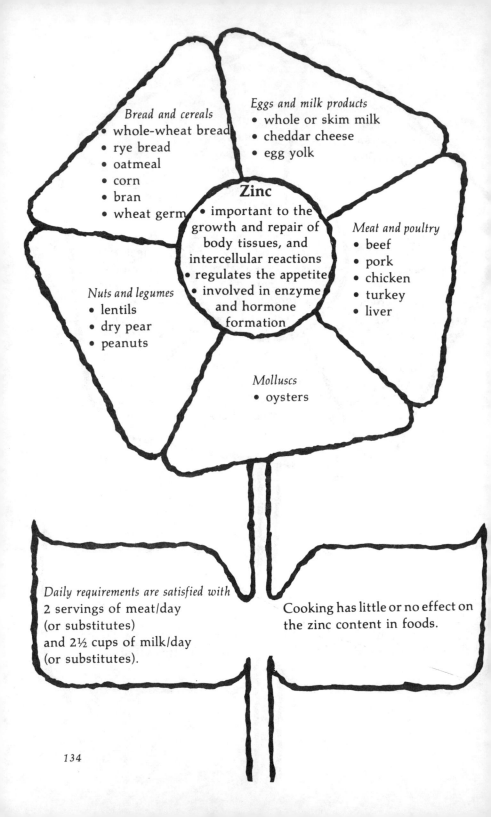

Bread and cereals
- whole-wheat bread
- rye bread
- oatmeal
- corn
- bran
- wheat germ

Eggs and milk products
- whole or skim milk
- cheddar cheese
- egg yolk

Zinc
- important to the growth and repair of body tissues, and intercellular reactions
- regulates the appetite
- involved in enzyme and hormone formation

Meat and poultry
- beef
- pork
- chicken
- turkey
- liver

Nuts and legumes
- lentils
- dry pear
- peanuts

Molluscs
- oysters

Daily requirements are satisfied with
2 servings of meat/day
(or substitutes)
and 2½ cups of milk/day
(or substitutes).

Cooking has little or no effect on the zinc content in foods.

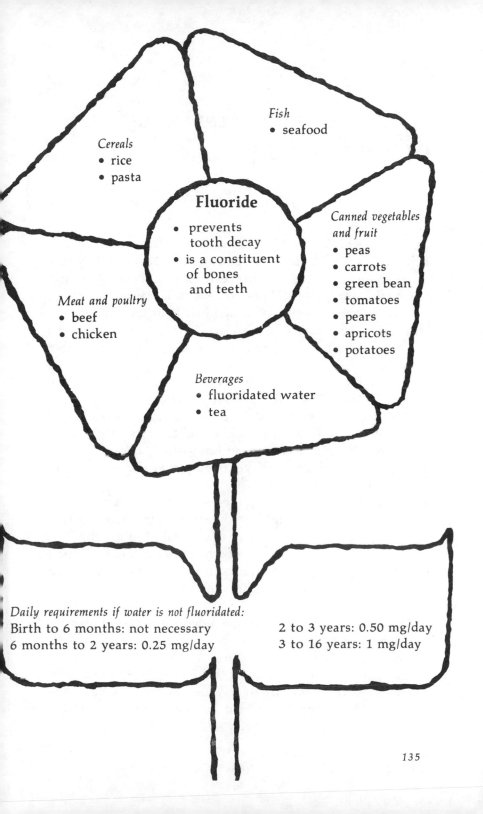

Fluoride

- prevents tooth decay
- is a constituent of bones and teeth

Cereals
- rice
- pasta

Fish
- seafood

Canned vegetables and fruit
- peas
- carrots
- green bean
- tomatoes
- pears
- apricots
- potatoes

Meat and poultry
- beef
- chicken

Beverages
- fluoridated water
- tea

Daily requirements if water is not fluoridated:
Birth to 6 months: not necessary
6 months to 2 years: 0.25 mg/day

2 to 3 years: 0.50 mg/day
3 to 16 years: 1 mg/day

CHAPTER TWELVE

A Child's Diet After Nine Months of Age

FEEDING A CHILD between nine months and six years of age never ceases to interest, if not torment, many parents! Poor parents! We have the uncanny knack of making mountains out of molehills. Unintentionally, we jeopardize the harmonious development of our child's healthy eating habits by misinterpreting his unpredictable behavior:

- "At six months, our child ate so well. Now at twenty months, he refuses to eat practically everything."
- "Mealtime is the most difficult time of my entire day."
- "My two-and-a-half-year-old daughter eats only peanut butter sandwiches day in and day out."
- "My three-and-one-half-year-old son would rather play with his food than eat it."
- "Mine refuses to eat vegetables. Any vegetables."

Surprising Fact — A child who eats too little arouses five times as much attention as one who eats too much.

Alarming Fact — Parents attach an importance to food which goes far beyond its true value; food is often used as a vehicle for reward and punishment, or as a means of bargaining!

- "If you don't finish your meat, you can't have any ice cream."
- "No dessert for you. You hit your sister."
- "Eat your green beans and you can have some dessert."

The "reward" foods are nearly always desserts, cakes, or candies. The foods "withheld as punishment" are also desserts, cakes, and candies.

This "sugar-pleasure-reward" association, reinforced by the child's environmental experiences, are bound to remain with him for a long time!

Important Fact — Healthful food attitudes are acquired around the table. Eating habits of parents have a tremendous influence on the child's own eating behavior.

A father who consistently refuses to eat broccoli, liver, and fish will have a hard time convincing his child to eat these foods. Can a mother who skips breakfast reprimand her children for wanting to do the same?

The pleasure a family experiences in eating a wide variety of foods is contagious and easily transmitted to a child. Inversely, new food experiences are rarely sought by a child brought up in an environment where food is perceived as a necessity and served in a routine and monotonous manner.

Without denying the preschooler's fluctuations in appetite, patience and understanding can help circumvent the problem. The acceptance of a few food whims is much better in the long run than daily confrontation around problem foods.

Respect for a child's appetite and the development of good eating habits begun in the early months of life must continue in spite of the odd problem encountered during the formative years. A better understanding of the total development of a child (physical growth, motor and social skills) will aid in the acceptance of appetite fluctuations.

Revealing Fact — The younger the child, the more willing he will be to try new foods, as a study conducted in the United States revealed. Seventy-seven percent of children between one and two years of age will try new foods. This percentage drops to 10% in children between two and four years of age, and to 7% in children four years of age and older.

A child who is taught to eat a variety of foods at a very young age will continue to derive much pleasure in diversifying his diet for the rest of his life.

It should be remembered that the preschooler's eating habits, his appetite fluctuations, and his whims, indicate on the one hand a slowing of his growth, and on the other hand an assertion of his personality and independence.

The Child's Point of View

A child wants to eat when he is hungry. Food brings him comfort and both physical and emotional satisfaction.

A child does not come into the world with eating habits already established. As we have seen previously, these habits are formed slowly but surely during the "first years of life."

Along with the food he eats, a child receives messages which enable him to shape his attitudes and feelings about the whole process of eating. A child who has been fed with love will "love to eat," but a child who has been fed with impatience and indifference will not have such a positive attitude toward his food. It is partly through his meals that a child makes contact with the outside world as it begins to play an ever-increasing part in his life. Toward the age of one, he begins to express his preferences clearly and reacts to the texture, temperature, taste, and color of his food, to the size of the helping he is given, and to the general atmosphere of the meal. If he refuses a dish, it is because one or more of these aspects displeases him.

His Tastes

Although no two children react in exactly the same way, common factors are nonetheless discernible in the pre-schooler.

Texture

He likes his food to be soft in consistency and not dry and hard. He really enjoys puddings which are runnier than usual, and cooked cereals which are less consistent; he prefers mashed potatoes to a baked potato, minced meat to steaks, and fresh bread to dry bread. These food preferences are due in part to the fact that at this age the child has little saliva, which normally would act as a lubricant.

Temperature

He likes to be served food which is "lukewarm," soup which has "cooled off," ice cream which has "softened," milk at room temperature, etc.

Flavor

He prefers mild flavors and he reacts to the slightest flavor changes — milk which is almost sour, and slightly over-cooked vegetables. Spicy and seasoned foods are unpopular, unless his cultural background encourages this type of dish. An Italian child will appreciate the flavor of garlic and onions more than his North American counterpart.

Color

He likes colors and color contrasts. A "bright" dish (chicken, carrots, and broccoli) produces a positive reaction, while a "dull" dish (fish, mashed potatoes, and yellow string beans) will not stimulate his appetite; to the contrary it might well deaden it! A child eats first with his eyes, more so than an adult. Colors fascinate him, whether they are on the plate or on the table: red place mats, striped napkins, a garnish of parsley on the potato, a green pepper ring on the tomatoes, a fruit salad of cantaloup and green grapes — there are so many ways of adding color to the table and pleasing the eyes of little ones.

Portion Size

Plates containing "miniature" portions get a better response from the child; one filled to the brim discourages him before he even starts. It is wiser to give him the pleasure of coming back for seconds than to force him to leave a half-filled plate. Food prepared in bite-size pieces is more appealing and easier to handle. A child must be given the chance to master the situation.

Mealtime Atmosphere

A calm and relaxed atmosphere helps the child to eat well. Loud "background" noise should be turned off at mealtime: the washer, the dryer, the fan, a blaring radio, the television set, etc. A child's attention cannot be split the same way as an adult's; he can only do one thing at a time. When noises or lively conversations are present at mealtime, he forgets to eat. A favorable atmosphere, on the other hand, encourages the acceptance of a new food.

Furthermore, the child likes to see what he is eating; he inspects his food. He will often pull a sandwich apart or break up a casserole simply to find out what foods are in it. He doesn't like mixtures. This is the "simple" food stage when food is easy to see, to handle, and to eat.

His Aptitudes

Knowing a preschooler's pattern of chronological motor, physical, and social development, enables us to better understand his eating behavior.

XII-1: The Preschooler's Motor and Social Aptitudes

Age	Manual Abilities	Physical and Social Behavior
6 to 12 months	• uses hands	• displays interest in texture and consistency • discovery through smell, handling
15 months	• grasps spoon, places it on the plate, but fills it improperly • holds spoon upside-down close to mouth	• slight decrease in appetite • everything goes into the mouth

	• often drops cup and spoon	
18 months	• drinks well from the cup but has difficulty putting it down • turns the spoon in his mouth	• growth rate slows • appetites decreases considerably • loves "rituals"
2 years	• drinks from a small glass held in one hand • puts spoon in mouth without turning it	• pulls objects apart and asks for help • learns to say "no" • begins to show whims and specific and monotonous preferences
3 years	• can pour liquids from a small container • rarely asks for help • uses a fork • makes little mess	• whims less apparent • more accommodating in his attitude
4 years	• uses a fork and a knife	• displays whims and goes on "hunger strikes" • able to set the table
5 years	• still prefers "simple" foods	• accepts new situations more readily • is influenced by others

His "Arrhythmical" Growth

During the first year of life, a child grows approximately 10 inches (25 cm), and triples his birth weight. It's a once-in-a-lifetime accomplishment! Throughout the preschool years, the child continues to grow but he adds only 16 to 17 inches (40 cm) to his height, and 23 pounds (10 kg) to his weight in the entire five years. After the first year, the yearly growth rate is about three to four inches (8 cm), and around four pounds (1.7 kg). The growth rate is slowing down.

XII-2: *A Child's Growth Rate*

	Birth	One Year	Six Years
BOYS			
height	20 in. (50 cm)	30 in. (75 cm)	46 in. (115 cm)
weight	7.5 lb. (3.3 kg)	23 lb. (10 kg)	45 lb. (19.8 kg)
GIRLS			
height	19 in. (48.5 cm)	29 in. (73.5 cm)	46 in. (115 cm)
weight	7.3 lb. (3.2 kg)	22 lb. (10 kg)	46 lb. (20 kg)

This obvious slowdown in growth is the reason for the preschooler's decrease in appetite. The eight-month-old baby who happily gobbles up everything in sight is growing at an almost visible rate, while the whimsical two-and-a-half-year-old hardly grows at all.

On the other hand, unexpected and unpredictable growth spurts account for the fluctuations in appetite during these early years. Suddenly the child grows in height, stops, puts on weight, then stops again. These intermittent growth "spurts" are accompanied by a temporary increase in appetite. Between these two growth spurts the appetite decreases. There is no need whatever to worry about this.

Despite these variations in his growth and appetite, the young child has special nutritional needs that must be met if the specific demands of his body are to be satisfied. The formation of his muscles, bones, and blood calls for an adequate consumption of foods rich in protein, calcium, phosphorus, vitamin D, and iron. Resistance to infections and the overall healthy functioning of the body necessitates adequate intake of foods rich in vitamins A, B, and C.

A varied, well-balanced diet is one of the keys to a child's health.

Food Choices at Different Ages

The preschooler adapts gradually to a varied diet and discovers new foods month after month. His diet is made up of basic foods which are prepared in various ways according to his capabilities. The evolution of the diet parallels the child's development, both physiologically and physically.

The following pages suggest a choice of foods adapted to various age groups and indicate the quantity to be consumed for each type of food.

Nine to Eighteen Months

Milk and milk products:
- from a glass: whole milk until 12 months and 2% milk after, if desired
- plain yogurt or fruit, for dessert
- cottage cheese or mild cheese, in certain dishes

Recommended quantity:
20 oz. (625 mL) of milk per day
(4 oz. (125mL) of yogurt or 3/4 oz. (22 g) mild cheese can replace 4 oz. (125mL) of milk)

Fruit and vegetables:
- cooked and mashed with a fork, except for ripe banana which can be eaten as is
- after 12 months, peaches and melons can be served raw; fruit juice, between 3 and 4 oz. (90 to 125 mL) per day

- avoid fruit with seeds: strawberries, raspberries, goose-berries, and red grapes

Recommended quantity:
Two small portions of fruit and vegetables per day

Meat, poultry, and fish:
- cut in bite-size easy-to-chew pieces
- ground meat, poached fish without bones, meatloaf

Recommended quantity:
1½ oz. (45 g) per day, approximately

Whole egg:
- after 10-12 months, the child can eat about four whole eggs per week, hard-boiled, poached, or scrambled.

Cereals:
- it is preferable that baby cereals be given and the type varied throughout the week
- occasionally offer oatmeal or cream of wheat and serve lukewarm

Recommended quantity:
7 tablespoons (105 mL) per day
whole-wheat bread, 1 slice per day or more

Snacking foods:
- bread crusts, a quarter of a peeled apple

Foods to be avoided:
- peanuts, nuts, potato chips since they can choke the young child, rich desserts, pastries and sweets since they tend to diminish the child's appetite and cause tooth decay

One-and-a-Half to Two Years

Milk and milk products:
- milk can be taken from a cup or incorporated into desserts, such as puddings, or taken in the form of yogurt, mild cheese, or cottage cheese with fruit

- whole milk, 2%, or skimmed, according to the needs of the child or doctor's orders

Recommended quantity:
20 oz. (625 mL) per day or its equivalent in milk products

Fruit and vegetables:
- cooked and finely cut, served with the greatest color contrasts
  Monday: carrots and broccoli
  Tuesday: cauliflower and fresh cherry tomato
  Wednesday: squash and asparagus
  Thursday: zucchini and green beans, etc.
- certain raw vegetables can exercise a baby's gums: carrot sticks, cauliflower flowerettes
- fruit is an excellent dessert and fruit juice may be served at snack time

Recommended quantity:
Two small portions of fruit and vegetables per day

Meat, poultry, and fish:
- meat cut into strips or bite-size pieces; pieces of fish, poultry or liver cut into small cubes; roasted meat cut into small pieces

Recommended quantity:
1½ - 2 oz. (45-60 g) per day

Whole egg:
- serve soft-boiled, poached, scrambled, or beat up in egg nog

Recommended quantity:
About four per week

Cereals:
- dry, or cooked, always served with milk

Recommended quantity:
½ cup (125 mL) per day
whole-wheat bread: one or two slices per day

Foods to avoid:
- fried foods, pastries, cakes, and cookies are unnecessary in the diet of a child of this age
- never give coffee, tea, or carbonated beverages to a child
- avoid hard-to-chew foods — peanuts, nuts, potato chips

Two to Five Years

The basic nutritional principles remain the same — a child eats all foods. Milk is incorporated into sauces or into desserts. Yogurt and cheese also provide calcium so essential in the building of a child's teeth and bones.

Whole fruit and vegetables are offered, either cooked or raw. Portions are increased gradually as the child grows older.

Meat is cut into pieces instead of minced; crisp bacon is also appreciated.

Candies, cakes, and pastries should not be part of the preschooler's diet. This concentrated source of calories satisfies his appetite but not his nutritional requirements and interferes with his acquisition of a varied and balanced diet.

Foods to avoid:
- fried foods and hard-to-chew foods — peanuts, nuts, and potato chips

Around five years of age

The child particularly rejects dishes prepared in sauces or as casseroles. Retain the basic foods: milk, vegetables, fruit, meat and cereals, served plain, without sauce or camouflaging. Children of this age prefer raw vegetables to cooked ones. The choice can, nevertheless, be large: green pepper rounds, sliced tomatoes, cauliflower flowerettes, lettuce-and-spinach salad, cole slaw and cubed apples, carrot salad and raisins, etc. The five-year-old is influenced by attitudes in his environment and by his friends' eating habits.

How much meat should a two-year-old be given? What is the correct serving size of fruit for a three-year-old?

It is very important to offer appropriate food portion sizes if the child's needs and appetite requirements are to be fulfilled. It is not enough simply to divide an adult portion in half.

A healthy child knows the amount of food he requires. This presupposes, however, that the child is offered healthy foods as part of his basic diet. The child given sweets and chocolates can easily lose control of his appetite, become a glutton, and end up with a good stomachache.

The table which follows indicates the approximate size of food servings suitable to a preschooler's appetite. They are very small but adequate enough to satisfy the nutritional needs of a child who eats a varied diet every day.

XII-3: *Suggested Portions from One to Six Years*

Food	1 year	2-3 years	4-6 years
Milk	½ cup (125 mL)	½ to ¾ cup (125 mL-180 mL)	¾ cup (180 mL)
Lean meat, poultry, fish	2 tablespoons (7 portions/ lb.)	3 tablespoons (6 portions/ lb.)	4 tablespoons (5 portions/ lb.)
Liver: once a week	2 tablespoons	3 tablespoons	4 tablespoons
Peanut butter	½ tablespoon	1 tablespoon	2 tablespoons
Egg	1	1	1
Orange juice or other juice rich in vitamin C	⅓ cup (90 mL)	½ cup (125 mL)	½ cup (125 mL)
Fruit, and yellow or green vegetables	2 tablespoons	3 tablespoons	4 tablespoons

Other vegetables (potatoes)	2 tablespoons	3 tablespoons	4 tablespoons
Other fruit	¼ cup	½ fruit	½ to 1 fruit
Bread	½ slice	1 slice	1½ slices
Dry cereal	⅓ cup (85 mL)	½ cup (125 mL)	½ cup (125 mL)
Cooked cereals, rice, macaroni, spaghetti	¼ cup (60 mL)	⅓ cup (85 mL)	½ cup (125 mL)

Food Preparation and Presentation

In order to stimulate a child's appetite, it is essential to offer him appetizing and easy-to-eat foods. It is very important to know how to prepare food properly so as to retain its color, flavor, texture, and nutritional value. Limp and discolored vegetables or dried-up and shrivelled pieces of meat will remain on a child's plate while a firm and colorful vegetable or a tender and juicy piece of meat is quickly eaten up!

Meats, Poultry, and Fish

The child enjoys these foods when they are juicy and tender, and easy to handle and chew.

The more tender cuts of meat, when gently cooked over low heat, will remain tender. The less tender cuts should be cooked longer in a small amount of liquid at a low temperature. Low heat and slow cooking will always help ensure tender and flavorful meat.

Liver, when cooked gently, maintains a good texture. Chicken livers are particularly tender and their mild flavor pleases a baby.

Meat or fish croquettes (tuna or salmon) or meatloaf, to which a larger than usual amount of liquid has been added, are popular with young children.

Poultry, which has been gently roasted (300°F to 325°F oven (150°C-170°C), 30 minutes per lb.), or simmered in a broth, produces equally tender and juicy, easy-to-chew meat, as long as it has been cut into small pieces before serving (remove small bones).

As for fish, slow-cooking over low heat preserves its fragile texture. Choose fish fillets or carefully remove all bones from fresh fish.

In all cases, lean cuts of meat and fish, fresh or frozen, should be selected. Serve in small pieces or in strips according to the child's abilities. One portion per day meets the nutritive needs of the preschooler.

Vegetables

Vegetables add color and vitamins to the main course. The right cooking procedure will help retain these important characteristics.

Never soak vegetables in water before cooking.

Cook vegetables in a small amount of boiling, salted water. Do not wait for the vegetables to change color or for them to become limp. Cut into small pieces or mash after cooking and serve immediately. Cooking vegetables in the pressure-cooker, or steam-cooking, also preserves their nutritive value as long as the cooking time does not exceed that indicated for each vegetable.

Retain the cooking water to later cook rice or cereals. A blended vegetable soup supplies both milk and vegetables to the child.

When the child is able to chew, he can experiment with a large choice of raw vegetables: carrots, green peppers, cauliflower, broccoli, turnip, celery, lettuce leaves, and cabbage.

Two small portions daily satisfy the needs of the pre-schooler.

Fruit

Children like the flavor of fruit. They eat fruits cooked at the beginning, and then raw, depending on the fruit and its characteristics. Apples in particular should be peeled until the child is three or four years old to prevent choking. Note that cooked fruit compotes of apples and pears, pears and peaches, prunes and apples, or just apples are very successful.

Serve unsweetened fruit to develop an appreciation for the real fruit flavor.

During the first two years, fruit containing small seeds, such as strawberries, raspberries, gooseberries, and grapes, should not be offered.

Dried fruit (prunes, dates, figs, raisins, apricots) can be cut up into small pieces as soon as the child chews properly (after two years). Supervise the child's tooth brushing after he has eaten these fruits since they can stick to his teeth.

Every day a child must eat a vitamin-C rich fruit. Oranges and grapefruits, or their juices, fresh or frozen, are among the best sources of this vitamin. Vitaminized apple juice or tomato juice are also rich in vitamin C.

Do not choose fruit drinks or "beverages" over fruit juices. These drinks are perhaps vitamin-C enriched, but do not contain the other nutrients found in real fruit juices.

Eggs

A whole egg is added to a child's diet toward the end of the first year (ten or twelve months) and is easily accepted by the child.

Hard-boiled eggs served in an egg cup, or cut up into a small plate and served with bread (fingers), pleases the most temperamental appetites. Poached or scrambled eggs may also be served with milk cheese.

An older child (three to six years) likes to bite into a hard-boiled or stuffed egg. Camouflaged in egg nog or in a custard, an egg always supplies good protein to the pre-schooler. A child can eat four eggs per week.

Bread and Cereals

This food group supplies protein, vitamins from the B-vitamin complex, iron, and calories at a bargain price. They are part of a well-balanced diet.

The young child (three to twelve months) enjoys the taste of precooked cereals. Later, he likes cooked cereals such as oatmeal and cream of wheat which have cooled, and later still, around the age of two, he crunches on dry cereals.

Publicity concerning dry cereals, presweetened, colored, or puffed often makes a choice difficult when selecting these foods. Actually, in the United States, 88% of mothers let their children choose their own favorite cereal, a type of freedom which can ruin a child's healthy eating habits. Whole-grain cereals *must* be selected since they retain all their nutritive qualities.

Some whole-grain cereals:
- hulled barley
- cracked wheat or bulgur

Cooked cereals:
- oatmeal
- cream of wheat
- wheat germ cereals
- muesli
- brown rice
- buckwheat
- millet

Dry cereals:
- muffets — plain and malt-flavored
- Weetabix
- Shredded Wheat (regular)
- Shredded Wheat (mini-wheats)
- Shreddies (presweetened)

A quarter cup (60 mL) of cooked cereal is equivalent to half a cup (125 mL) of dry cereal, or half a slice of whole-wheat bread.

A child with a small appetite is nourished more quickly when served cooked cereals. Always serve milk with cereal in order to reap the maximum nutritive benefits. The nutritive value of cooked cereals can be increased by replacing the water used in cooking by milk or by adding powdered milk to the cereal before cooking.

They can be naturally sweetened with dry fruit (raisins or prunes) or with fresh fruit (one-half a banana or small seasonal fruits). Add little or no sugar.

Pasta is part of this food group. It supplies less nutrients than cereal or bread. Combined with cheese, milk, eggs, meat, or vegetables, it provides variety to a meal and supplies energy.

Milk and Milk Products

This last-but-not-least important food group plays a primary role in the growth of the child. Few foods possess comparable nutritional qualities.

By the time the baby is six months old, he can start drinking whole milk. Skim and 1% milk is not recommended for children before the age of twelve to eighteen months because of its high protein concentration and low caloric value. Between one to six years of age, the child must receive the equivalent of two-and-a-half cups (625 mL) of milk daily. If it is not all taken in liquid form, water or fruit juices must be provided to quench a child's thirst. Carbonated beverages or sweetened fruit "drinks" are to be avoided.

A child prefers milk at room temperature, which means that milk should be removed from the refrigerator some time before mealtime.

Around six months, he begins to drink from *a cup with a spout* which facilitates the transition from bottle to glass. Towards the middle of the second year, a child can handle a cup well. To avoid spills, the cup is offered at the end of the meal.

Around age two, the child drinks from a glass; a small but wide glass is easier to handle than a taller but narrower one. It is not necessary to fill it to the brim.

Around age three, a child is able to pour the milk with the help of a small container or pitcher. He is happy to master this technique and this may encourage him to drink a bit more milk.

At this age, an occasional straw can perform miracles. In order to increase the nutritional value of the preschooler's diet, it is recommended that milk be incorporated into soups, sauces, and desserts. Other milk products can replace the liquid milk, such as mild cheeses, yogurt, ice cream, and ice milk:

- 6 oz. (180 mL) of milk (preschooler's portion)
- 1 oz. (30 g) of milk cheese
- 6 oz. (180 mL) of yogurt
- ¾ cup (180 mL) ice cream
- ¾ cup (180 mL) ice milk

A child must not be fed ice cream exclusively as a milk substitute under the pretext that he does not drink milk. Ice cream contains more calories than milk and might lead to an overweight problem. Ideally, ice cream can serve as a substitute on special occasions. Chocolate milk is not a good substitute for milk. It contains more calories, more sugar, and promotes a bad habit.

Mealtime Atmosphere

Timetable

Regular mealtimes promote better food consumption in the preschooler; a child eats better when fed at regular intervals. If mealtime is too late, a tired child will not eat. Breakfast takes place usually half an hour after rising, the midday meal at noon, and the night meal at six o'clock. The evening meal can be later if a snack is provided around four o'clock.

Physical comfort at mealtime

For a child to sit down at the dinner table only to find that he has his nose at table level, that the chair rocks, that his feet do not touch the floor, or that he has to eat with oversized utensils, are factors which detract from his enjoyment of eating.

An uncomfortable child usually eats less than one who is comfortable at the dinner table.

A minimum of comfort prevents many unfortunate situations:
- high chair, with foot support
- a table suited to his needs
- smaller utensils
- good bib
- small but wide unbreakable glass, half-filled
- bowl, or convex plate rather than a flat one
- a little decor stimulates appetites
- colorful tablecloth or place mats
- centerpiece, a few dried or fresh flowers
- lit candle for a special supper meal

Child's participation

Around the age of three, a child is able to help his mother and loves to feel useful. Active participation at meal-preparation time improves his attitudes toward foods and can even stimulate his appetite. Rather than having to be dragged to the table, he will sit willingly, proud of his "adult" accomplishments such as:
- setting the table
- placing serviettes at each place setting
- pouring milk or juice into unbreakable glasses
- placing raw vegetables or biscuits in to a plate (unbreakable)
- placing bread into a bread basket.

Accidents and spills are inevitable. An understanding mother accepts them calmly and continues to ask for a child's help. An opposite reaction may create a lack of self-confidence in a child.

As a child grows, the types of tasks increase as well. He learns to:
- butter bread
- stuff celery sticks
- break eggs for father's omelette
- hull peas, husk corn.
- His self-satisfaction grows as his responsibilites multiply.

Snacks

We live in an age of "coffee breaks," or snacks at any time during the day. Unfortunately it is often difficult to associate snacking with nutrition. Many favorite foods at snacktime supply empty calories and suppress the appetite for the important foods served at mealtime. This phenomenon also affects the eating habits of the child; continual nibbling at cookies, sweets, and potato chips stuffs the child with calories without nourishing him and prevents him from consuming foods at mealtime which are more nutritious.

A child's need for snacks

A child will snack according to his individual needs. Snacks are useful to complete the child's nutritional needs, but they should not replace meals. They must help satisfy the body's requirements but not become a social need! If this fact is kept in mind, the adult can easily forego snacks. On the other hand, the young child eats small amounts at any given time and rapidly uses up his reserves. He is unable to go long periods without eating.

The week-old baby requires small quantities of milk, six or seven times per day. His ability to consume larger and larger amounts of food develops gradually. Around the age of ten months, he eats three or four times a day. His meals are larger, and the interval between meals is longer. Between the ages of six months to six years, a normal child who eats a good breakfast around eight in the morning, can go until noon easily without problems. An afternoon snack is often necessary and does not affect the evening meal as long as it is a "healthy snack."

The three-year-old to five-year-old child who gets up early, eats breakfast rapidly, and spends the morning in a nursery school, benefits from a ten o'clock snack. Experiments conducted with small children showed that fruit juice was sufficient. Fruit juices are rich in vitamins and minerals, are easily digested, do not cause allergies, and furnish quick energy in record time.

Consider the case of a child who is all wound up at mealtime and has difficulty swallowing even half or a quarter of the food given to him. He would certainly benefit from nutritive snacks which would fill his nutritional gaps. Care must be taken, however, since this strategy carries its own risks. The child can easily get into the habit of eating between meals rather than at mealtime.

It is thus impossible to set fixed rules with regards to snacks. The following general guidelines may help a mother decide whether or not her child does or does not need a snack and help guide her as to the correct choices:

- a child who eats like a bird at mealtime, will eat even less if snacks are offered. Snacks could therefore be the cause of a lack of appetite at mealtime.
- a "healthy" snack offered two to two-and-a-half hours before the next meal does not affect a normal child's appetite.
- the amount given at snacktime must be controlled in order to prevent this light meal from becoming a heavy one.
- the food chosen for snacks is of prime importance. It must complete and not detract from the nutritional needs of the child.

Criteria for a "healthy" snack

For a child, a healthy snack should:
- attract the eye and satisfy the palate. It is pleasant to look at and good to eat
- satisfy but not fill up
- supply valuable nutrients (vitamins, minerals), but not contain empty calories
- vary from day-to-day
- keep the mind and the fingers busy
- allow the child's participation in its preparation

Ideas and Recipes for Snacks

A. Snacks rich in vitamins and minerals, but poor in calories

Unsweetened fruit juices (4 to 6 oz. (124 to 180 mL))
- apple, grape, pineapple, tomato, orange, grapefruit, cranberry, watermelon juices*
- apricot or prune nectar
- "two-fruit" drink (orange and banana juice)*

NOTE: These fruit juices may also be frozen in popsicle containers, and are a popular and refreshing treat during the summer.

Fresh fruit
- apple, quartered, cut in rings, or as apple sauce
- apricots
- whole or sliced banana
- fresh cherries
- fresh coconut, cubed
- fruit "kebabs"*
- orange or grapefruit, in segments
- seedless green grapes, in a small bunch
- melon cubes (cantaloup, honeydew, or watermelon)
- peach or pear pieces
- prunes
- ripe strawberries, blueberries, raspberries
- mandarin oranges

Dried fruit (more concentrated in calories and sugar; brush teeth well after eating)
- raisins
- figs
- dates

Raw vegetables
- avacado cubes
- green cabbage, quartered
- carrot sticks
- flowerettes of cauliflower or raw broccoli
- celery
- celery stuffed with peanut butter or seasoned cottage cheese
- cucumber sticks or slices
- green peas in their pods
- green pepper rings
- cherry tomatoes
- turnip sticks
- zucchini slices
- vegetable "kebabs"

B. More Nutritional Drinks (for active children, with a large appetite)

- banana milk*
- orange milk*
- "peanut" milk*
- grape juice and lime*
- milk, ice cream, and banana* (or strawberries)
- prune-juice shake*

C. More Nutritional Snacks (for active children, with a large appetite)

- nut or fruit bread, with cheese spread,* or served plain
- cheese cubes
- cheese sticks
- fruit and cheese (apple and cheese) "kebabs"
- muffin
- squirrel crunch*
- cheese and vegetable (celery and cheese) "kebabs"
- plain or fruited yogurt

*Recipes on the following pages.

RECIPES

Watermelon Drink

Ingredients
Juice of half a lemon or lime
1 cup (250 mL) orange juice, fresh or frozen reconstituted
4 cups (1 L) of large pieces of watermelon, with seeds removed
Preparation
1. Place all ingredients into the blender and blend well.
2. Strain if necessary (if seeds have fallen into the juice).
3. Serve cold.
Yield
5 cups (1.25 L) of juice
Comments
Watermelon supplies a certain amount of vitamins A and C

"Two-Fruit" Drink

Ingredients
1 cup (250 mL) orange juice
1 small banana or ½ cup (125 mL) strawberries
Preparation
1. Place the two ingredients into the blender and mix well.
2. Serve very cold.
Yield
2 child-sized portions

Fruit "Kebabs"

Ingredients
2 small bananas, cut into pieces
10 to 12 large strawberries
2 oranges, quartered
Preparation
1. Thread the fruit onto 4 bamboo or wooden skewers, alternating banana, strawberry, and orange sections
2. Keep in the refrigerator, if necessary.
3. Eat as soon as possible to prevent the banana from discoloring.
Yield
4 "kebabs"
Comments
Pitted prunes may be used instead of strawberries, peaches instead of oranges, or let the child concoct his own "kebabs."

Banana Milk

Ingredients
1 cup (250 mL) ripe bananas, cut in small pieces
½ teaspoon (2 mL) vanilla
1 cup (250 mL) 2% milk
Preparation
1. Place the two bananas and the milk into the blender and mix well
2. Add the vanilla.
3. Refrigerate and serve cold.
Yield
2 to 3 child-sized portions

Orange Milk

Ingredients
1 quart (1.2 L) 2% milk (5 cups)
1 6¼-oz. (180 mL) container of frozen, concentrated orange juice, unsweetened
Preparation
1. Place ingredients into the blender and mix well.
2. Refrigerate and serve cold.
Yield
6 cups (1.5 L)
Comments
This drink may be kept several days in the refrigerator.

"Peanut" Milk

Ingredients
4 cups (1 L) of 2% milk
⅓ cup (85 mL) smooth peanut butter
1 tablespoon (15 mL) honey (optional)
Preparation
1. Place peanut butter into the blender.
2. Add a small amount of the milk and mix well.
3. Add remaining milk gradually, mixing constantly. Add honey. Mix well.
4. Refrigerate. Stir gently before serving.
Yield
4 cups (1 L)

Grape Juice and Lime

Ingredients
4 oz. (125 mL) grape juice, unsweetened
1 scoop lime sherbert
Preparation
1. Put the two ingredients into the blender; blend for 30 to 40 seconds.
2. Taste and enjoy.
Yield
2 small glasses or 1 generous portion
Comments
Another version: 4 oz. (125 mL) apple juice and 1 scoop orange sherbert is equally successful with children and adults alike.

Milk, Ice Cream, and Banana (or Strawberries)

Ingredients
1 cup (250 mL) 2% milk
1 scoop vanilla ice cream
1 banana, very ripe, cut into pieces
Preparation
1. Place ingredients into the blender and mix well.
2. Serve very cold.
Yield
2 child-sized portions
Comments
A festive snack for special days! The banana may be replaced by
½ cup (125 mL) fresh or frozen unsweetened strawberries.

Prune-Juice Shake

Ingredients
1 cup (250 mL) milk
4 cooked prunes, pitted
¼ cup (60 mL) prune juice
Preparation
1. Place all ingredients into the blender and mix well.
2. Serve cold.
Yield
2 child-sized portions
Comments
Excellent for gently relieving constipation.

Cheese Spread (on fruit, nut, or rye bread, etc.)

Ingredients
1 cup (250 mL) cottage cheese
½ cup (125 mL) crushed pineapple, unsweetened
Preparation
1. Place ingredients into the blender and mix well.
2. Store in refrigerator and spread on bread just before serving.
Yield
1 cup (125 mL).
Comments
½ cup apricot, apple, or peach puree may be used in place of the
pineapple (125 mL).

Squirrel Crunch

Ingredients
4 cups (1 L) quick-cooking oatmeal
1 cup (250 mL) shredded coconut
1 cup (250 mL) finely chopped walnuts
1 cup (250 mL) wheat germ
1 cup (250 mL) sunflower seeds
⅓ cup (85 mL) honey
⅓ cup (85 mL) corn oil
½ teaspoon (2 mL) vanilla

Preparation
1. Set oven at 350°F (180°C).
2. Mix the first five ingredients in a large bowl.
3. Heat the honey and add to dry ingredients; add oil and vanilla. Mix with wooden spoon or hands.
4. Place mixture on well-greased cookie sheets. Cook for 30 minutes, stirring once during cooking. Cool.
5. Store in hermetically sealed containers. Keep in a cool place.

Yield
8 cups (2 L) of cereal

Comments
After cooking, raisins or chopped dates may be added. This cereal is very nourishing. Serve only a small portion (¼ to ⅓ cup or 60 to 85 mL) so as not to spoil the child's appetite.

Evaluation of Eating Habits

The formation of a child's eating habits begins in the cradle and continues throughout the preschool years, from birth to six years of age, and a finicky six or seven-year-old is likely to stay this way all his life.

Good or bad habits are acquired in the family home — not at the neighbor's! From the age of six or seven years old, the family influence decreases and exterior influences play a more dominant role — school, friends, the neighborhood snack bar, and so on.

A child who is accustomed to eating good food will be less inclined to adopt nutritional habits which are more or less injurious to his physical development and his health. A child who has never learned proper eating habits will be more easily attracted to coffee and doughnuts for breakfast, french fries and soft drinks for lunch, and pizza and chocolate milk for supper!

Before the age of six, the situation can still be corrected. The following questionnaire will enable you to evaluate the quality of your child's eating habits. Put a checkmark under the appropriate "yes" or "no" answer.

The results are calculated according to the directions shown at the end of the questionnaire.

XII-4: *Evaluation of a Child's Eating Habits*

	YES	NO
1. He eats breakfast every morning.	___	___
2. He snacks on whatever is available throughout the morning instead of eating breakfast.	___	___
3. He drinks milk at every meal or consumes an equivalent milk substitute (see: "Food choices at different ages" in this chapter).	___	___
4. He only drinks fruit-flavored "drinks" or carbonated beverages.	___	___
5. He refuses all vegetables.	___	___
6. He enjoys cooked and raw vegetables and eats them at every meal.	___	___
7. He drinks orange juice every day or eats another food rich in vitamin C (see: previous chapter: "Vitamin C").	___	___

	YES	NO
8. He recognizes and likes whole-grain cereals. He eats them every day.	——	——
9. He systematically refuses to try new foods.	——	——
10. He eats fruits as long as they have been sweetened.	——	——
11. He eats liver at least once a week or some other food rich in iron.	——	——
12. He recognizes and likes beef, lamb, pork, and poultry.	——	——
13. He has never tasted fish.	——	——
14. He enjoys mealtime.	——	——
15. For snacks, he eats cookies or candies.	——	——
16. He can control his appetite and knows when to stop eating.	——	——
17. He recognizes and likes at least three varieties of fish.	——	——

How to Calculate Your Score

- Score ten points for each "yes" answer to questions 1, 3, 6, 7, 8, 11, 12, 14, 16, 17.

- Deduct ten points for each "yes" answer to questions 2, 4.

- No points are awarded for any of the other "yes" answers.

Points Obtained	Quality of Eating Habits
100	Excellent
80-100	Good
60-80	Acceptable
40-60	Improvement is desirable
0-40	It's time to do something about it!

CHAPTER THIRTEEN

The Transitional Diet —
Nine to Eighteen Months

THE TRANSITIONAL DIET corresponds to a form of
feeding which is adapted to the physiological and physical
capabilities of the nine to eighteen-month-old child. It is
called "transitional," since the texture of the food is more
consistent than purees eaten prior to this period, but softer
than the foods eaten after this period. The flavors of the
foods are also milder, less spicy, and less-seasoned than
what will normally be served once the child is eighteen
months old.

Vegetables are cooked the same way as described in the
recipes for purees, then mashed with a fork after cooking.
Meats, poultry, and fish are not blended for as long, or are
simply minced, or cut into small pieces according to a baby's
feeding skills. Fruit can be served pureed or cooked,
mashed with a fork, or offered in stewed form. Some raw
fruits are introduced at this time such as melon and cantaloup. Bread can be served toasted, plain, cut in strips or
fingers, or in muffin form as well. Rusks are also popular
at this age.

The child's appetite gradually decreases after the age of
one year since the rapid-growth period is over. For this
reason, suggested portions are quite small, but they take
into account the nutritional needs of a child of this age.

XIII-1: *Suggested Portions from Nine to Eighteen Months*

Baby cereals: 7 tablespoons (105 mL)
                                 mixed with about ¾ cup
                                 (180 mL) milk

Fruit juice:	3 to 4 oz. (90 to 125 mL)
Vegetables and meat dinners:	¼ cup (60 mL)
Fish:	1½ oz. (45 grams)
Vegetables:	2 tablespoons (30 mL)
Stewed fruit:	¼ cup (60 mL)
Whole-wheat bread or muffin	½ slice (occasionally 1 whole slice for vegetarians)
Vegetable soup:	3 oz. (90 mL)
Whole milk:	4 oz. (125 mL)
Cottage cheese:	¼ cup (60 mL)
Cheese cubes:	1 oz. (30 gm)
Yogurt:	3 oz. (90 mL)
Jellied fruit dessert:	¼ cup (60 mL)

Feeding Schedule

- a child of this age adopts the family's timetable and eats three meals a day and one snack
- he drinks from a cup, eats some foods with his fingers
- on certain days he wants to be fed, at other times he chooses to eat by himself
- around twelve months of age, he starts to use a spoon
- at this age there is no room in the child's diet for rich desserts, pastries, and sweets
- avoid hard-to-chew foods, peanuts, nuts and potato chips

SEVEN MEAT AND SEVEN VEGETARIAN MENUS

Transitional Menus

With Meat	**Vegetarian**
1. orange juice	1. orange juice
barley baby cereal with milk	barley baby cereal with milk
whole milk	whole milk
beef, rice, and vegetables*	rice, vegetables, and cheese*
apple sauce*	apple sauce*
whole-wheat bread	whole-wheat bread
whole milk	whole milk

soft-boiled egg
bread fingers
¼ peach cut in small pieces
whole milk

snack: whole milk

2. apple juice
oatmeal baby cereal with
milk
whole milk

poached fish in milk*
pureed potato and carrot
whole-wheat bread
¼ ripe banana, mashed
whole milk

cottage cheese
pureed prunes and apples*
whole-wheat bread
whole milk

snack: whole milk

3. orange juice
mixed baby cereal with milk
whole milk

chicken with rice and
vegetables*
whole-wheat bread
¼ pear, mashed
whole milk

vegetable potage
bread fingers
small cube of cheese
¼ ripe banana, mashed
whole milk

4. apple juice
oatmeal baby cereal with
milk
whole milk

soft-boiled egg
bread fingers
¼ peach cut in small pieces
whole milk

snack: whole milk

2. apple juice
oatmeal baby cereal with
milk
whole milk

pureed vegetables and
legumes*
whole-wheat bread
¼ ripe banana, mashed
whole milk

cottage cheese
pureed prunes and apples*
whole-wheat bread
whole milk

snack: whole milk

3. orange juice
mixed baby cereal with milk
whole milk

lentils, rice, and vegetables*
whole-wheat-bread
¼ pear, mashed
whole milk

vegetable potage
bread fingers
small cube of cheese
¼ banana, mashed
whole milk

4. apple juice
oatmeal baby cereal with
milk
whole milk

surprise liver and beef loaf*
mashed zucchini
whole-wheat bread
cantaloup in small pieces
whole milk

snack: whole milk

"two-cheese" macaroni*
pureed apricots
whole milk

snack: whole milk

legume surprise*
mashed zucchini
whole-wheat bread
cantaloup in small pieces
whole milk

snack: whole milk

"two-cheese" macaroni*
pureed apricots
whole milk

snack: whole milk

5. orange juice
soya baby cereal with milk
whole milk

pureed pork and leeks*
whole-wheat bread
apple sauce
whole milk

poached egg
asparagus in small pieces
½ slice whole-wheat bread
jellied fruit dessert*
whole milk

snack: whole milk

5. orange juice
soya baby cereal with milk
whole milk

vegetables au gratin*
whole-wheat bread
apple sauce
whole milk

poached egg
asparagus in small pieces
½ slice whole-wheat bread
jellied fruit dessert*
whole milk

snack: whole milk

6. apple juice
rice baby cereal with milk
whole milk

chicken and rice
green beans in small pieces
pureed apples and pears*
whole milk

cream of carrots*
(see cream of vegetable soup)
corn bread muffin
peach yogurt
whole milk

snack: whole milk

6. apple juice
rice baby cereal with milk
whole milk

rice and cheese
green beans in small pieces
pureed apples and pears*
whole milk

cream of carrots*
(see cream of vegetable soup)
corn bread muffin
peach yogurt
whole milk

snack: whole milk

7.	orange juice	7.	orange juice
	soya baby cereal with milk		soya baby cereal with milk
	whole milk		whole milk
	poached fish*		lentils, rice, and vegetables*
	pureed green vegetables		whole-wheat bread
	whole-wheat bread		stewed apricots
	puree of prune and apple*		whole milk
	whole milk		
	soft-boiled egg		soft-boiled egg
	cooked julienne carrots		cooked julienne carrots
	whole-wheat bread		whole-wheat bread
	¼ frosty banana*		¼ frosty banana*
	whole milk		whole milk
	snack: whole milk		snack: whole milk

*Recipes available in this book — see recipe index

XIII-2: *Nutritive Value of the 7 Transitional Menus with Meat*

Meat menus are calculated according to the suggested portions

Day	Calories	Protein (g)	Calcium (mg)	Iron (mg)	Vit. B12 (Ug)	Vit. C (mg)
1	857	43	1050	18.9	4.2	70
2	822	47	733	15.7	3.2	58
3	908	49	1219	17.8	3.0	75
4	914	58	759	20.1	3.3	78
5	823	47	1049	16.9	4.0	89
6	882	38	1218	18.6	3.0	58
7	903	54	1131	18.5	3.0	75
Daily average						
	872[1]	56[2]	1022	18[3]	3.3	72[4]
Quantities Recommended:						
Canada	1100-1300	18-20	500	6	0.3-0.4	20
U.S.A.	945-1300	18-23	540-800	15	1.5-2	35-45

1. The average number of calories is below that recommended by Recommended Nutrient Intakes for Cana-

dians and the Recommended Dietary Allowances (U.S.) but is close to the amount actually consumed by six to ten-month-old babies. Once more, these recommendations are considered to be quite generous, and could benefit from a slight reduction in the recommendation for calories. For babies older than eleven months, it is easy to increase the calories simply by increasing the size of servings according to the child's appetite.

2. In spite of the small servings of meat or fish, the entire menu supplies more than twice the quantity of required protein. Milk also contributes to the protein intake.

3. The major source of iron comes from baby cereals. It would be difficult to satisfy an infant's requirements for iron without them.

4. By eating a varied menu consisting of small amounts of fruit, vegetables, and fruit juice, the infant easily meets his vitamin C requirements without having to resort to vitamin supplements.

XIII-3: *Nutritive Value of the 7 Vegetarian Transitional Menus*

Vegetarian menus include milk products and eggs

Day	Calories	Protein (g)	Calcium (mg)	Iron (mg)	Vit. B12 (Ug)	Vit. C (mg)
1	826	38	1107	17.6	3.7	67
2	865	42	735	16.2	3.0	56
3	908	39	1226	17.4	2.8	72
4	855	40	764	16.6	3.0	74
5	873	45	1093	17.3	4.0	93
6	902	38	1324	17.6	3.0	58
7	879	44	1104	17.5	3.0	78

Daily average

	872[1]	40[2]	1050	17.1[3]	3.2	71

Quantities Recommended:

Canada	1100-1300	19-21	500	6	0.3-0.4	20
U.S.A.	945-1300	15-23	540-800	15	1.5-2	35-40

1. Despite the absence of meat, poultry, and fish, a vegetarian child can easily meet his caloric and protein

requirements by eating a varied diet such as the one proposed.

A vegan child who does not eat any milk products or eggs would benefit from a longer period of breast-feeding and foods such as tofu, baby cereals, and pureed legumes added to the fruit and vegetables in order to complete his nutritional needs. A vitamin-B12 supplement· should also be taken since foods of vegetable origin do not supply this vitamin at all.

2. Protein requirements are slightly higher in the vege-tarin menu in order to conform to the recommendations of the W.H.O. (F.A.O.)

3. The major source of iron comes from baby cereals. They are an important part of the young vegetarian child's diet and should not be replaced prematurely by cereals destined for the older child or adult, even if these are whole-grain cereals.

RECIPES

Beef, Rice, and Vegetables

Ingredients
1 lb. (500 g) lean minced beef
1 teaspoon (5 mL) butter or margarine
½ cup (125 mL) converted rice[1]
1 cup (250 mL) vegetable cooking liquid and water
1½ cups (375 mL) vegetables, finely cut

- ¾ cup (180 mL) fresh tomatoes, peeled and chopped, plus ¾ cup (180 mL) onions, green peppers, and finely chopped celery.
- ½ cup (125 mL) finely chopped celery, plus ½ cup (125 mL) diced carrots, plus ½ cup (125 mL) green peas.
- ½ cup (125 mL) fresh tomatoes, plus ½ cup (125 mL) finely chopped celery, plus ½ cup (125 mL) cut green string beans or any other favorite vegetable.

Preparation
1. Bring water and cooking liquid to a boil; add rice. Lower heat and cook for approximately 10 to 15 minutes.

2. In another saucepan, fry meat gently in melted fat. Add 1½ to 2 cups (375 to 500 mL) water, half-cooked rice, and selected vegetables. Bring to a boil. Reduce heat and simmer until vegetables are tender.
3. Take from heat and cook slightly.
4. Empty into small containers (¼ cup (60 mL)) and freeze.

Yield
3 cups (750 mL)
1 child-sized serving before 1 year: ¼ cup (60 mL)

Storage Life
10 to 12 weeks

1. Such as Uncle Ben's.

Rice, Vegetable, and Cheese Casserole

Ingredients
½ cup (125 mL) white sauce, medium thickness[1]
½ cup (125 mL) cooked rice (brown or converted)
½ cup (125 mL) pureed vegetables (asparagus, carrots, zucchini, or squash)
6 tablespoons (90 mL) grated cheddar cheese

Preparation
1. Mix all ingredients together.
2. Freeze in individual portions of ¼ cup (60 mL) each or refrigerate a few days until ready to serve.
3. Heat in double-boiler or use the method described in "two-cheese" macaroni to reheat.
4. Before serving, add 1 teaspoon (15 mL) shredded cheese on top of each portion.

Yield
1½ cups (375 mL) or 6 portions of ¼ cup (60 mL)

Storage Life
3 to 4 weeks in the freezer

1. Recipe described on page 174.

Poached Fish in Milk

Ingredients
1 to 2 fillets or salt-water fish steaks (sole, cod, ocean, perch, haddock, salmon) — 8 oz. or 240 g
1 to 2 tablespoons (15 to 30 mL) finely chopped onions
¼ to ½ cup (60 to 125 mL) whole milk

Preparation
1. Pour ¼ cup (60 mL) milk into a frying pan and heat gently. Add onion. Cook several minutes.
2. Add fish fillets or steaks. Cover and cook over low heat 5 to 10 minutes or until the fish becomes white (or light pink, as in the case of salmon), and it flakes when tested with a fork.
3. Remove from heat and flake entire fish with fork removing all bones, if necessary.
4. Divide into portions (1½ oz. or 45 g) and place into small aluminum containers with a small amount of milk and onions. Cover with aluminum foil and freeze or serve one portion immediately, storing the remainder in the refrigerator for a few days.
5. Reheat in a 400°F (205°C) oven for about 10 minutes.

Yield
5 containers of portions of 1½ oz. (45 g)

Storage Life
4 to 6 weeks

White Sauce

Ingredients
2 tablespoons (30 mL) butter, oil, or margarine
2 tablespoons (30 mL) flour
½ cup (125 mL) whole milk
½ cup (125 mL) chicken stock or vegetable cooking liquid

Preparation
1. Melt fat in saucepan.
2. Add flour and mix well. Cook a few minutes.
3. Gradually add liquids, stirring constantly until the sauce thickens. Cook one additional minute.

4. Cool and store in refrigerator or use immediately in a recipe.

Yield
1 cup (250 mL)

Storage Life
About 3 to 4 days in refrigerator
About 4 weeks in freezer

Pureed Legumes and Vegetables

Ingredients[1]
1 cup (250 mL) cooked legumes (dried peas, red kidney beans, soya beans, etc.), pureed either in a blender, in a food processor, or with a food mill.
½ cup (125 mL) pureed green or yellow vegetables
1 cup (250 mL) white sauce, medium thickness[2] (still warm)

Preparation
1. To the warm white sauce, add pureed legumes and vegetables. Mix well.
2. Divide into portions of about ¼ cup (125 mL) and empty into small aluminum containers for freezing or simply store in the refrigerator for a few days.
3. Reheat in double-boiler at serving time.

Yield
2½ cup (625 mL) or 10 portions of ¼ cup (60 mL)

Storage Life
4 to 6 weeks

1. Ingredients may be divided by half or by thirds so that smaller quantities can be produced.
2. Recipe described on page 174.

Chicken with Rice and Vegetables

Ingredients
½ chicken, 2-3 lb. (1 to 1.3 kg) cut into three or four pieces
1 teaspoon (5 mL) finely chopped parsley
Water

2 tablespoons (30 mL) minced onion
3 carrots, peeled and cut into coins
1 stalk of celery cut in pieces
1 cup (250 mL) green peas or green string beans, fresh or frozen
½ to ⅔ cup (125 to 170 mL) converted rice, uncooked

Preparation
1. Place chicken and parsley in saucepan. Bring to a boil, reduce heat, and simmer 15 minutes.
2. Add celery, onion, and carrots and simmer 10 minutes longer.
3. Add the cup of green vegetables, fresh or frozen, and rice, and cook an additional 30 minutes or until all ingredients are tender.
4. Remove from heat. Take out chicken and debone carefully.
5. Place half the chicken and ½ cup (125 mL) of the cooking liquid into the blender. Blend and empty into a large bowl; blend the rest of the chicken in the same way.
6. Place the rice and vegetables and 1½ cups (375 mL) of the bouillon into the blender; blend and empty into a large bowl; stir the mixture, empty into containers and freeze.

Yield
About 3 cups (750 mL) or 12 portions of ¼-cup (60 mL) each

Storage Life
10 to 12 weeks

Comments
This preparation can be made without a blender when the child is able to chew on regular food.

Lentils, Rice, and Vegetables

Ingredients
½ cup (125 mL) cooked lentils, mashed or pureed[1]
¼ cup (60 mL) brown rice, cooked[2]
½ cup (125 mL) white sauce, medium thickness[3]
¼ cup (60 mL) green or yellow vegetables, cooked and finely chopped

Preparation
1. Reheat white sauce slightly.
2. Add lentils, rice, and vegetables, and mix well
3. Cool and store in refrigerator or empty into small freezer containers of about ¼ cup (60 mL) for the freezer.

Yield
1½ cups (375 mL) or about 6 portions of ¼-cup (60 mL) each

Storage Life
3 to 4 weeks in freezer
2 to 3 days in refrigerator

1. Any other legume may replace lentils.
2. A white converted rice may replace the brown rice, if preferred.
3. Recipe described on page 174.

Cream of Vegetable Soup

Ingredients
½ cup (125 mL) milk
¼ to ½ cup (60 to 125 mL) raw vegetables (carrot coins or cauliflower flowerettes, asparagus or green string beans cut in pieces)
½ slice of whole-wheat bread
1 teaspoon (5 mL) butter or margarine

Preparation
1. Cook vegetables in small amount of water.
2. Place cooked vegetables, cooking liquid, milk, bread, and butter into the blender.
3. Blend for about 30 seconds.
4. Reheat and serve.

Yield
1½ cups (375 mL) or 4 3-oz. (90 g) portions

Storage Life
1 month

Comments
These cream soups supply the child with two important foods at the same time: milk products and vegetables. They can be accompanied with a mild cheese and rusks.

Surprise Liver and Beef Loaf

Ingredients
1 lb. (500 g) chicken livers (or beef or lamb)
1 medium onion, quartered
1¼ lb. (626 g) lean minced beef (blade or round)
⅔ cup (170 mL) uncooked oatmeal (rapid-cooking)
1 cup (250 mL) tomato juice
1 egg
½ teaspoon salt (after age one)

Preparation
1. Preheat oven to 350°F (180°C).
2. Place the well-cleaned, raw liver, and the onion, quartered, into the blender. Blend until a smooth puree is obtained.
3. In a large bowl soak the oatmeal in tomato juice for about 10 minutes; add the puree of liver, minced meat, egg, and salt, and mix well.
4. Empty into a well-greased loaf pan. Cook 60 to 75 minutes.
5. Remove from heat and let sit 5 minutes before slicing. Cut into small pieces for babies between 6 and 18 months or slice for older children.

Yield
16 servings or more for children 6 to 18 months
8 to 10 servings for children between 3 and 6 years

Storage Life
10 to 12 weeks in freezer
3 days in refrigerator

Legume Surprise

Ingredients
1 cup (250 mL) cooked white or red kidney beans
2 teaspoons (10 mL) corn oil
3 tablespoons (45 mL) minced onion
¼ cup (60 mL) kernel corn (pureed, if baby is not able to chew)
1 teaspoon (5 mL) tomato paste
1 tablespoon (15 mL) water

Preparation
1. Puree cooked legumes in a blender or food processor.
2. Mix water and tomato paste together.
3. Fry onion in oil. Add pureed legumes, diluted tomato paste, and kernel corn.
4. Cook over low heat until well mixed and hot.
5. Serve immediately if desired or store in refrigerator for several days.
6. This preparation can also be frozen in small freezer containers and reheated at the last minute.

Yield
Approximately 1 cup (250 mL) or 4 portions of ¼-cup (60 mL) each

Storage Life
2 to 3 days in the refrigerator
4 to 6 weeks in the freezer

Two-Cheese Macaroni

Ingredients
2 cups (500 mL) cooked macaroni, blended with ¾ cup (180 mL) milk
2 eggs
1 cup (250 mL) milk
1 cup (250 mL) cottage cheese
4 to 6 tablespoons (60 to 90 mL) grated cheese (parmesan, cheddar)
2 teaspoons (10 mL) butter or margarine
½ teaspoon (2 mL) salt (after 1 year)

Preparation
1. Beat eggs in blender; add milk, cottage cheese, grated cheese, salt, and the butter or margarine.
2. Add cooked "blended" macaroni. Mix well.
3. Place mixture in small individual aluminum containers. Cover with aluminum foil. Label and freeze.
4. To serve, remove from freezer and cook in 350°F (180°C) oven for about 40 minutes.

Yield
3 cups or 12 ¼-cup (60 mL) portions

Storage Life
4 to 6 weeks

Comments
This macaroni contains less calories than the conventional dish since cottage cheese is used; consequently, it has a milder flavor. It can be cooked immediately after preparation in a 350°F (180°C) oven, for 30 minutes.

Pureed Pork and Leeks

Ingredients
5 to 6 oz. (150 to 180 g) cooked roast pork, fat removed
1 large leek
½ cup (125 mL) cooking liquid from vegetables

Preparation
1. Cook the leek. Save the green part for soups and use only the white part in this recipe.
2. Cut pork into small pieces, cut up leek, and add to blender along with vegetable cooking liquid. Blend.
3. Empty into freezer tray and freeze.

Yield
8 to 10 cubes: 1 serving represents ¼ cup (60 mL)

Storage Life
10 to 12 weeks

Comments
Any lean cooked meat plus one cup of vegetables and vitamin-rich vegetable juice can constitute a similar meal.

Vegetables au Gratin[1]

Ingredients
1 cup (250 mL) white sauce, medium thickness[2]
1 cup (250 mL) cooked carrots, mashed or pureed
1 cup (250 mL) green vegetable, pureed (broccoli, green peas, asparagus)
⅓ cup (85 mL) grated mozzarella cheese

Preparation
1. Gently reheat white sauce. Add cheese and let it melt by stirring a few minutes.
2. Add vegetables and mix well.
3. Cook and pour into small freezer containers and refrigerate until ready to serve.
4. Reheat in a double-boiler before serving.

Yield
3 cups (750 mL) or 12 ¼-cup (60 mL) portions

Storage Life
2 to 3 days in the refrigerator
4 to 6 weeks in the freezer

1. All quantities may be decreased if a smaller quantity is preferred
2. Consult white sauce recipe on page 174.

Jellied Fruit Dessert

Ingredients
1 package of unflavored gelatine
¼ cup (60 mL) cold water
½ cup (125 mL) boiling water
8 oz. (250 mL) juice
8 oz. (250 mL) fruit puree (optional)

Preparation
1. Pour cold water into a medium bowl. Sprinkle gelatine over water and allow to soak.
2. Add boiling water and dissolve gelatine.
3. Add fruit juice, mixing well.
4. Add pureed fruit and mix well.
5. Pour into small individual bowls, if desired.
6. Refrigerate for a few hours and serve when gelatine is firm.

Yield
11 2-oz. (30 mL) portions

Suggestions
• unsweetened grape juice (undiluted Welch's) with pureed pears

- apple juice with pureed peaches or pureed banana
- frozen, diluted orange juice with pureed, frozen, sieved strawberries

NOTE: For purees, any unsweetened, canned-in-its-own-juice fruit may be used, except pineapple, which prevents the gelatine from setting.

CHAPTER FOURTEEN

The Preschooler's Menu — Eighteen Months to Six Years

AROUND THE AGE of eighteen months, a child is usually ready to eat the same foods as other members of the family. His "particular needs" must not be forgotten, however: simple foods, easy-to-eat, served lukewarm or at room temperature, in small portions.

The eighteen-month-old child does not have a big appetite; his growth has slowed down. To perk up his interest in healthy foods, imagination and ingenuity must be used:

- Give your dishes amusing names: Peter Rabbit Salad, Crunchy Muffin, Mystery Soufflé, Pink Surprise.

- Make the food look as attractive as possible: animal-shaped sandwiches, fruit salads arranged in the form of funny faces, a nest of vegetables; use color and texture contrast.

- Keep mealtime a happy time. As mentioned previously, the atmosphere which prevails at the dinner table can stimulate a child's appetite or make it disappear!

- Vary the setting occasionally. Picnics in the park, on the balcony, or in the backyard can help stimulate the appetite.

- Invite a friend to lunch: company stimulates appetites. All of these suggestions are applicable to a child up to the age of six.

Seven Menus

1. *Breakfast*
   Grapefruit cut in sections
   Crunchy Muffins*
   6 oz. (180 mL) milk

   Lunch
   Little Red Hen Salad*
   Slice of bread
   Pink Surpise*
   6 oz. (180 mL) milk

   Dinner
   Small bacon omelette
   Asparagus tips
   Rusk or toast, cut into
   triangles
   Peach Ambrosia*
   6 oz. (180 mL) milk

2. *Breakfast*
   Orange juice
   Golden Soufflé*
   6 oz. (180 mL) milk

   Lunch
   Homemade fish sticks*
   "Nest" of mashed potato
   filled with sliced carrots,
   and sprinkled with parsley
   Apple sauce
   6 oz. (180 mL) milk

   Dinner
   "Super-Duper"*
   Rusk with cubes of mild
   cheese
   Cantaloup balls and
   seedless white grapes
   6 oz. (180 mL) milk

3. *Breakfast*
   Magic Breakfast*
   Slice of toast or a brioche

   Lunch
   Mother Hubbard Soufflé*
   Grated cabbage salad
   Funny Banana Bread*
   6 oz. (180 mL) milk

   Dinner
   Meat-Loaf Surprise*
   Zesty Zucchini*
   "Happy Apple"*
   6 oz. (180 mL) milk

4. *Breakfast*
   Orange cut in sections
   Oatmeal and dried fruit
   6 oz. (180 mL) milk

   Lunch
   Chicken-and-egg casserole*
   Cherry tomatoes
   Slice of bread
   Homemade yogurt* and
   fruit in season
   6 oz. (180 mL) milk

   Dinner
   Thin slice of ham on
   buttered bread, cut into
   strips
   Sailboat Salad*
   Frosty Banana*
   6 oz. (180 mL) milk

5. *Breakfast*
   Fruit Velvet*
   Hot roll or muffin

Lunch
Tuna Delight with
Cucumber Super-Sauce*
"Peter Rabbit Salad"*
"Apple Snow"*
6 oz. (180 mL) milk

Dinner
Small croquette of minced
beef
"Nest" of mashed potato
filled with finely chopped
green beans
Slice of bread
Chinese Pears*
6 oz. (180 mL) milk

6. *Breakfast*
Wake-Up Breakfast*
Slice of toast or a brioche
6 oz. (180 mL) milk

Lunch
"Hide and Seek" (with
chicken livers)*
Broccoli flowerets and
carrot coins
Mashed potato
Sunshine Fruit*
6 oz. (180 mL) milk

Dinner
Macaroni cheese
Fairy Salad*
Super-Strawberry*
6 oz. (180 mL) milk

7. *Breakfast*
Vitamin-enriched apple
juice
Boiled egg
Bran muffin
6 oz. (180 mL) milk

Lunch
Little Red Riding Hood
Special (quartered
tomatoes and celery sticks)
Salmon Mousse
Popsifruits*
6 oz. (180 mL) milk

Dinner
Chicken in sauce, in a "nest"
of rice sprinkled with
parsley
Squash, cut into cubes
6 oz. (180 mL) milk
Bamboula Mousse*

*Recipes available in book, consult index.

RECIPES

Crunchy Muffin
Ingredients
1 English muffin
¼ cup (60 mL) of grated cheddar cheese

Preparation
1. Cut muffin in half horizontally and sprinkle each half with
   cheese.

2. Place the halves under the broiler for a few minutes, until cheese has melted.

Yield
2 small portions

Little Red Hen Salad

Ingredients
½ cup (125 mL) grated carrots
1½ oz. (45 g) cooked chicken, cut into cubes
2 tablespoons (30 mL) finely-chopped celery or green pepper
1 to 2 tablespoons (15-30 mL) mayonnaise

Preparation
1. Gently mix all the ingredients together.
2. Arrange them in the shape of a nest on the plate.
3. Garnish with a sprig of parsley.

Yield
1 portion

Pink Surprise

Ingredients
4 oz. (125 mL) plain yogurt
¼ cup (60 mL) crushed strawberries, unsweetened
1 teaspoon (5 mL) honey (optional)

Preparation
Mix the ingredients together, and serve

Yield
1 portion

Peach Ambrosia

Ingredients
3 peaches, peeled and cut into small pieces
1 sliced banana
1 tablespoon (15 mL) lemon juice
1 tablespoon (15 mL) light brown sugar
¼ cup (60 mL) grated coconut

Preparation
1. Cut the pieces of peach and banana onto a dessert plate.
2. Sprinkle them with the lemon juice, then sift on the brown sugar and grated coconut.
3. Serve cold.

Yield
4 small portions

Golden Soufflé

Ingredients
12 eggs
1 lb. (500 g) creamed cottage cheese
6 slices of whole-wheat bread
Maple syrup or honey

Preparation
1. Heat the oven to 350°F (180°C).
2. Put the eggs and the cottage cheese in the blender and blend to a smooth consistency.
3. Arrange the slices of bread in a well-greased ovenproof dish.
4. Pour the egg and cheese mixture over the bread and bake for 30 minutes, or until the eggs are firm and golden.
5. Serve with maple syrup or honey.

Yield
6 adult portions, or 12 child-sized portions

Remarks
This recipe can very easily be reduced to half or a third of the quantities given above merely by using a smaller baking-dish. Golden Soufflé makes an excellent breakfast on Saturdays or Sundays. If served for lunch or dinner, it provides the child with a light nourishing meal.

Homemade Fish Sticks

Ingredients
1 lb. (500 g) filleted white fish (bass, sole, haddock)
½ cup (125 mL) toasted wheat germ
¼ cup (60 mL) sesame seeds
1 teaspoon (2 g) salt

½ teaspoon (2 mL) paprika
2 small eggs
2 tablespoons (30 mL) corn oil

Preparation
1. Grease a cookie sheet or other shallow oven-proof dish. Heat the oven to 350°F (180°C).
2. Place the fish fillets on a chopping-board and cut them into sticks 1 in. (2.5 cm) wide by 4 in. (10 cm) long.
3. Mix the wheat germ, sesame seeds, salt and paprika in a bowl.
4. Beat the eggs in another bowl, pour in the corn oil and whisk with a fork.
5. Roll each piece of fish in the wheat germ mixture, then soak it in the egg mixture. Roll it once more in the wheat germ mixture, then place it on the greased pan.
6. Cook in the oven for about 15 minutes.
7. Serve hot with homemade sauce tartare, a green salad and purée baked potatoes.

Yield
4 adult portions or 8 child-sized portions

Remarks
This recipe is very popular with children. It is a good way of giving them fish with all its nutritive qualities intact.
The wheat germ and the sesame seeds may be replaced with whole wheat cereals, well crushed.

"Super-Duper"

Ingredients
1 lb. (500 g) small zucchinis (3 or 4), washed and sliced
1 cup (250 mL) homemade chicken bouillon
1 teaspoon (2 g) salt
⅛ teaspoon basil (a pinch)
⅛ teaspoon thyme (a pinch)
½ teaspoon marjoram (a pinch)
2 cups (500 mL) milk

Preparation
1. Bring the chicken bouillon and salt to a boil in a saucepan, then add the zucchini, cover the saucepan and simmer until the zucchini slices are soft (about 5 to 10 minutes).

2. Let the mixture cool a little, then add the basil, thyme and marjoram.
3. Put everything in the blender and reduce to puree.
4. Pour the puree back into the saucepan and add the milk gradually; reheat, but do not bring to a boil.
5. Serve in soup bowls, with a spoonful of plain yogurt on top if desired.

Yield
6 child-sized portions

Magic Breakfast

Ingredients
1 egg
4 oz. (125 mL) orange juice (either fresh, or frozen juice reconstituted)
2 oz. (60 mL) milk

Preparation
1. Put all the ingredients into the blender and mix for about 30 seconds.
2. Serve.

Yield
1 portion

Remarks
This breakfast is quickly prepared — and quickly gobbled up!

Mother Hubbard Soufflé

Ingredients
1 cup (250 mL) grated Canadian cheese — about 4 oz. (120 g)
2 tablespoons (30 mL) butter
4 tablespoons (60 mL) all-purpose flour
¼ teaspoon (1 mL) dry mustard
½ 6-oz. (180 g) can of tuna, well drained
5 egg yolks
5 egg whites
1 cup (250 mL) hot milk

Preparation
1. Preheat the oven to 375°F (190°C).

2. Place first 7 ingredients into the blender. Blend 15 seconds.
3. Pour mixture into saucepan and cook over low heat until thick and smooth.
4. Beat egg whites until firm, but not dry, then gently fold into first mixture.
5. Pour into well-greased 1½-quart (1½-L) mold. Bake in oven about 30 minutes.

Yield
4 child-sized portions

Comments
This "super soufflé" never fails — children love its soft texture.

Funny Banana Bread

Ingredients
1½ cups (375 mL) whole-wheat flour
2 teaspoons (10 mL) baking powder
½ teaspoon (2 mL) baking soda
½ teaspoon (2 mL) salt
1 cup (250 mL) natural bran
¼ cup (60 mL) walnuts, chopped
¼ cup (60 mL) sunflower seeds
1 egg, slightly beaten
¼ cup (60 mL) honey
¼ cup (60 mL) corn oil
¼ cup (60 mL) skim milk
3 to 4 ripe bananas, mashed

Preparation
1. Mix first four dry ingredients together; add bran, nuts, and sunflower seeds.
2. In another bowl, mix beaten egg, oil, milk, and bananas in the blender or food processor a smooth mixture is obtained.
3. Add this last mixture to dry ingredients and mix well.
4. Pour into oiled bread pan.
5. Cook in 350°F (175°C) oven for about 1 hour.

Yield
1 loaf

Comment
It is simply delicious and I suggest that the recipe be doubled so that reserves are available! Thick slices may be individually frozen and thawed in desired amounts.

Zesty Zucchini

Ingredients
2 lb. (1 kg) zucchini
1 8-oz.-can (240 g) tomato sauce
½ cup (125 mL) grated cheese
salt, pepper, and oregano

Preparation
1. Preheat oven to 350°F (180°C), and grease an oven-proof dish.
2. Wash zucchini, and cut into thin slices; do not peel.
3. Place a layer of zucchini into dish and season with seasonings; place a second layer, and season again.
4. Mix the tomato sauce and oregano, and pour over zucchini.
5. Sprinkle with cheese and cover dish.
6. Cook about 25 minutes.

Yield
6 portions

Freezer Storage life
3 months

Happy Apple

Ingredients
4 apples
4 teaspoons (20 mL) honey
4 tablespoons (60 mL) grated coconut
Lemon juice

Preparation
1. Heat the oven to 350°F (180°C).
2. Core the apples and cut them in two.

3. Put them in an oven-proof dish or on a sheet of aluminum foil, sprinkle each half with honey and coconut, then sprinkle with lemon juice.
4. Cover the dish, wrap it in aluminum foil.
5. Bake in the oven for 20 to 30 minutes.

Yield
4 portions or 8 half portions

Chicken and Egg Casserole

Ingredients
¾ slice whole wheat bread, crumbled
¼ cup (60 mL) milk
1½ cups (375 mL) chicken, cooked and diced
1 tablespoon (15 mL) chopped onion
¼ teaspoon (60 mL) salt
1 tablespoon (15 mL) chopped parsley
2 tablespoons (30 mL) corn oil
1 egg + 1 egg yolk

Preparation
1. Heat the oven to 350°F (180°C).
2. Soak the bread in the milk, then add the chicken, onion, salt, parsley, and oil.
3. Beat the egg yolks and add them to the mixture.
4. Beat the egg white until stiff, then fold it carefully into the mixture.
5. Pour the mixture into an oven-proof dish, and stand this in a cakepan with hot water in it.
6. Cook for about 30 minutes, or until the center of the mixture has set. Then remove the dish from the oven, and serve.

Yield
4 portions

Homemade Yogurt

Ingredients
5 cups (1.2 L) 2% milk
¼ cup (60 mL) powdered skim milk
¼ cup (60 mL) plain yogurt

Preparation
1. Mix milk and the milk powder together.
2. Heat mixture to boiling (180°F [82°C]); check the thermometer.
3. Remove mixture from heat and cool to 113° to 116°F (46°C) (this will take about 20 minutes).
4. Place yogurt into a large pyrex or earthenware bowl. Gradually add milk and mix well.
5. Cover bowl with Saran Wrap or aluminum foil; wrap bath towel around it to keep heat in and shield it from draughts).
6. Place bowl in a warm place where the temperature does not go above 150°F (65°C); (a warm oven with temperature turned off and checked with thermometer, near a radiator, or in a warm room where there are no draughts).
7. Let mixture set for 5 to 12 hours. Do not disturb bowl. The warmer the place, the quicker the yogurt will form. In a cooling oven, it will take about 8 to 10 hours — or overnight. As soon as the yogurt has set, refrigerate immediately. Use this yogurt in the preparation of recipes which follow.

Comments
Yogurt preparation is simple but delicate. Temperature must be kept properly maintained to guarantee success

Yield
5 cups (1.2 L)

Storage life
1 month

Sailboat Salad

Ingredients
1 small cantaloup
2 slices of packaged Swiss or Canadian cheese
Lettuce, washed, well drained, cut into strips
4 toothpicks

Preparation
1. Place lettuce into the bottom of 4 bowls.
2. Quarter cantaloup, remove seeds, and place each quarter on a bed of lettuce.

3. Cut cheese slices diagonally, then use toothpicks as "masts" to hold the triangles of cheese (the "sails") and stick them into the cantaloup quarters.
4. Serve with cold meats.

Yield
4 portions

Frosty Banana

Ingredients
1 peeled banana
2 tablespoons (30 mL) plain yogurt
2 tablespoons (30 mL) grated coconut or finely chopped nuts

Preparation
1. Cover banana with yogurt.
2. Roll in coconut or chopped nuts.
3. Place "frosty" banana on a dessert plate and serve.

Yield
1 portion

Fruit Velvet

Ingredients
¾ cup (180 mL) plain yogurt
½ 6¼-oz. (180 mL) can frozen grape juice or frozen orange juice

Preparation
1. Place ingredients into blender, and blend to milkshake consistency.
2. Serve.

Yield
2 to 3 4-oz. (125 mL) portions

Comments
Simply delicious.

Tuna Delight

Ingredients
1 6-oz. (180 g) can tuna
1 egg beaten

¼ cup (60 mL) milk
1 tablespoon (15 mL) vegetable oil
¼ cup (60 mL) chopped onion
1 tablespoon (15 mL) finely chopped parsley
½ teaspoon (1 mL) basil

Preparation
1. Preheat oven to 425°F (220°C).
2. Mix together: egg, milk, oil, onion, parsley, and basil.
3. Flake tuna with a fork and mix it with the other ingredients.
4. Pour mixture into a small oven-proof dish.
5. Bake in the oven for about 25 minutes.

Yield
4 child-sized portions

Freezer Storage Life
3 months

Comment
To round off this seafarer's meal, accompany with Cucumber Super-Sauce.

Cucumber Super-Sauce

Ingredients
1 small cucumber, grated, with or without peel
½ teaspoon (2 mL) chopped onion
¼ cup (60 mL) mayonnaise
1 tablespoon (15 mL) finely-chopped parsley
¼ cup (60 mL) plain yogurt
1 tablespoon (15 mL) lemon juice

Preparation
1. Throughly mix all ingredients and serve with fish.

Yield
¾ cup (180 mL)

Comment
A guaranteed winner!

Peter Rabbit Salad

Ingredients
¼ cup (60 mL) grated carrot
¼ cup (60 mL) grated cabbage
1 tablespoon (15 mL) mayonnaise

Preparation
1. Mix all ingredients together, and serve.

Yield
1 portion

Apple Snow

Ingredients
1 cup (250 mL) unsweetened apple sauce
2 egg whites
1 tablespoon (15 mL) honey
1 tablespoon (15 mL) grated lemon rind

Preparation
1. Place ingredients into the blender and beat to the consistency of whipped cream.
2. Serve in small individual bowls.

Yield
4 to 6 portions

Chinese Pears

Ingredients
4 ripe pears
2 oz. (60 g) finely chopped walnuts
4 teaspoons (20 mL) honey
1 teaspoon (5 mL) cinnamon or ginger

Preparation
1. Preheat the oven to 350°F (180°C).
2. Peel and core pears; place in oven-proof dish.
3. Mix together nuts and honey.
4. Stuff centers of the pears with the honey and finely chopped nuts mixture.

5. Sprinkle with cinnamon or ginger.
6. Cook for about 30 minutes, or until the pears are soft.
7. Serve either hot or warm.

Freezer Storage Life
3 to 5 months

Wake-Up Breakfast

Ingredients
1 cup (250 mL) fresh or frozen reconstituted orange juice
1 cup (250 mL) fresh strawberries or quartered peaches
2 eggs
½ cup (125 mL) powdered skim milk
½ cup (125 mL) water

Preparation
1. Place all ingredients into the blender and blend thoroughly.
2. Serve.

Yield
4 to 6 child-sized portions

Freezer Storage Life
6 weeks

Comment
This is a complete breakfast in a glass!

"Hide and Seek" with Chicken Livers

Ingredients
4 slices of bacon
4 chicken livers

Preparation
1. Set the oven to "broil."
2. Cut chicken livers and slices of bacon in half.
3. Wrap each piece of liver in a strip of bacon and secure it with a toothpick.
4. Place under the broiler for about 8 minutes, or until the bacon is crisp. Turn once during cooking.
5. Remove from the oven, take out the toothpicks and serve.

Freezer Storage Life
3 months

Comment
When I saw my daughter eating her "Hide and Seek" with obvious relish, I said to her, "So now you like liver, do you?" "No, Mom," she replied, "it's the bacon I like."

Sunshine Fruit

Ingredients
2 pears
2 bananas
12 unsweetened strawberries, either fresh or frozen
1 cup (250 mL) plain yogurt
1 teaspoon (5 mL) cinnamon
A few chopped nuts

Preparation
1. Peel and core pears; cut into pieces.
2. Peel and slice bananas.
3. Wash and dry the strawberries, and cut them in half.
4. Mix together the fruit, yogurt and cinnamon and refrigerate for at least 1 hour.
5. Sprinkle with chopped nuts and serve.

Yield
6 child-sized portions

Comment
Seedless grapes may be substituted for the strawberries.

Fairy Salad

Ingredients
1 apple, grated, with or without peel
¼ cup (60 mL) raisins
1 tablespoon (15 mL) mayonnaise

Preparation
1. Mix together all ingredients, and refrigerate.
2. Serve on a lettuce leaf.

Super-Strawberry

Ingredients
1 envelope unflavored gelatin
¼ cup (60 mL) cold water
¼ cup (60 mL) boiling water
1 6¼-oz. (180 mL) can frozen concentrated orange juice, unsweetened
1 6¼-oz. (180 mL) can container cold water
1 cup (250 mL) unsweetened fresh or thawed strawberries

Preparation
1. In large bowl sprinkle gelatin over ¼ cup (60 mL) cold water, and let soak for 5 minutes.
2. Pour ¼ cup (60 mL) boiling water over gelatin mixture and mix well until gelatin has dissolved.
3. In blender, blend strawberries, undiluted orange juice concentrate, and container of cold water.
4. Blend until smooth.
5. Pour the pureed strawberry and orange mixture into gelatin mixture. Mix well.
6. Refrigerate a few hours until firm.

Yield
6 portions

Popsifruits

Ingredients
2 cups (500 mL) plain yogurt
1 6¼-oz. (180 mL) can of fruit juice, unsweetened and undiluted
Popsicle sticks and molds

Preparation
1. Pour yogurt into a bowl. Thicken in freezer for about 1 hour.
2. Pour undiluted frozen fruit juice into blender together with the half-frozen yogurt, and blend until smooth.

3. Pour the mixture into popsicle molds, push a popsicle stick into each mold, and freeze.
4. To serve, run very hot water over the molds to loosen the popsicles.

Yield
10 popsicles

Comment
Try orange juice, grape juice, pineapple juice — they are all delicious, for children and adults alike.

Bamboula Mousse

Ingredients
1 cup (250 mL) cooked pitted prunes
3 ripe bananas
½ teaspoon (2 mL) almond extract
¼ cup (60 mL) grated coconut (optional)

Preparation
1. Place all ingredients into the blender, blend until smooth.
2. Mix in the grated coconut.
3. Serve.

Yield
4 to 6 child-sized portions

Freezer Storage Life
3 to 5 months

CHAPTER FIFTEEN

A Few Special Problems

Whims

1. What to do with a child who refuses to eat?

TO BEGIN WITH, it is not unusual to find a preschooler on a "hunger strike." But what causes this behavior? If the child simply refuses to eat at mealtime but stuffs himself between meals with foods which do not provide any nutrients, but are sufficient in calories to fill him up, by the end of the day there will be a serious lack of protein, calcium, and vitamins.

If this situation persists for any length of time, the reasons must first be found in order to arrive at the solution.

Generally speaking, a refusal to eat is a behavioral problem which goes beyond the context of the meals themselves; it is a reaction to the general attitude of the child's parents. He is reacting perhaps because he was forced to finish his bottle as a baby, or was overfed during his first few years. He finds it easy to do so since he has become less hungry; he also feels the need to assert himself; he seeks attention; he realizes that his refusal to eat worries his parents so he starves himself to win attention and get his own way.

What not to do:

- force the child to remain at the table until his plate is empty

- promise dessert if he finishes what is on his plate
- serve leftovers from the last meal on the same plate for his next meal
- make him eat "one bite for Daddy — and one for Mommy — and one for Grandma," and so on
- talk about the nutritional content of the food; i.e., foods which make you grow, good for the hair, etc.

What to do:

- calmly accept food refusal
- do not show disapproval, or concern, either visibly or verbally
- if the child is hungry between meals, explain gently but firmly that the next meal is coming soon. Do not tell him that he is hungry because he missed the last meal.
- avoid speaking about food, vitamins, or food likes or dislikes at the table
- be prepared to see your child go hungry for a few days. He will acquire better eating habits as a result.
- give him the extra attention he is looking for — but between meals!

2. Will the growth of a child be stunted if he refuses to drink milk?

Milk and milk products are very important during a child's growth. They play an important role in teeth and bone formation and are very difficult to replace as no other food group possesses the same nutritive qualities. The child can grow, but his bones and teeth may grow more slowly and be formed weakly.

Why does a child refuse to drink milk? is it too hot? Too cold? Is the glass too big? The following recommendations may prove helpful.

Serving Milk
Serve milk in a smaller, colorful glass . . . with a straw. A three-year-old child can serve himself from a small jug.

Setting an Example

The child is first and foremost an imitator! If parents drink milk at mealtime, the example they set is far more effective than verbal encouragement. If extra calories and un-satured fats are a problem for the parents, skim milk can easily be chosen instead.

Camouflaging It

Should the child consistently refuse to drink milk, he might prefer to "eat" his milk. At breakfast give him hot cereals cooked in milk. At noon, offer him yogurt or a scoop of ice cream for dessert. For supper, serve his meat, poultry, or fish in a white sauce, or give him a cream of vegetable soup with cubes of mild cheddar cheese (see substitutes).

Dressing It Up

Milk goes down smoothly if its taste is disguised. Try serving milk mixed with fruit juice, or a "superdrink" made with yogurt and fruit juice. Do not add honey, sugar, or chocolate to the milk (consult snack recipes).

3. Can vegetables be replaced in the preschooler's diet?

Vegetables are often the "problem" food since mothers usually insist they be eaten. Forcing a child to finish his vegetables will probably reinforce his dislike.

Before removing them from his diet, try to find out why he dislikes them.

a) Do the parents like vegetables and eat a large variety regularly?

Where food tastes are concerned, the parents' eating patterns and their influence on the child should never be underestimated. The father's food preferences, in particular, have a great bearing on the eating habits of his children. If he dislikes broccoli, carrots, or asparagus, his children will usually refuse to eat them too. If he enjoys eating them, the children will imitate him.

The way in which vegetables are prepared and served

plays an important role in their acceptance. Overcooked, colorless vegetables without texture or taste will no doubt be rejected. A well-cooked vegetable, tender but firm, brimming with taste and color, and served in a small quantity, is far more easily accepted.

The child who was initiated early as an infant or before the age of two to a variety of vegetables flavors will be more likely to accept vegetables later on as well.

b) Has the mother tried all the vegetables available before giving up?

A mother should not be discouraged after one food refusal. Perseverance is the key to acquiring healthy eating habits. A vegetable which is usually refused suddenly becomes appetizing when servd with a favorite dish.

c) Raw vegetables are usually more popular with children.

This is an advantage because vitamins and minerals are preserved and the cellulose fiber found in vegetables is responsible for the proper functioning of the intestines. One more reason for them to be included in a child's diet — they can be eaten at mealtime or as a snack. Here are a few examples: lettuce and spinach salad, green pepper and cucumber rings, cherry tomatoes, cauliflower rosettes, carrot and celery sticks, and grated cabbage and carrot salad.

If a mother has tried everything and the child still persists in refusing both cooked and raw vegetables, another source of vitamins, minerals and cellulose must be found. Nature thinks of everything. Fortunately fruit possesses almost the same nutritive qualities as vegetables. The two vegetable portions a child must consume daily can temporarily be replaced by two fruit portions.

The fruit family offers many variations in color, taste, and nutritive values. A child will benefit more if a fruit rich in vitamins and minerals is chosen. Some of the best ones are: cantaloup, strawberries, citrus fruit (oranges and grapefruit), fresh or dried apricots, peaches, prunes, watermelon. Reconstituted frozen fruit juices (orange, grapefruit and grape) are good sources of vitamin C. Apricot and prune nectar supply also vitamin A and iron. Fruit-flavored drinks enriched with vitamin C are not recommended.

4. If a child refuses to eat meat, can it be replaced with equally nutritious foods?

When a child systematically refuses to eat a food, I would suggest you reread the first section of this chapter.

Meat is not indispensable in the child's diet. It can be replaced by other equally good protein sources, such as poultry, fish, eggs, or cheese. However, every time you remove a food from a child's diet, you run the risk of making it more monotonous. One ounce (30 g) of meat can be replaced by:

- 1 oz. (30 g) fish, fresh or canned
- 1 oz. (30 g) poultry
- 1 oz. (30 g) cheese, such as cheddar
- 1 egg
- ¼ cup (60 mL) cottage cheese
- 6 oz. (180 mL) yogurt
- 6 oz. (180 mL) milk
- ½ cup (125 mL) cooked legumes (beans, lentils, dried peas)

A child who eats neither meat or organ meats (liver, heart, kidney) should be given molluscs (oysters, clams, scallops), dried peas (white beans, lima beans, navy beans), dried fruits, whole-grain cereals, and green vegetables in order to obtain a sufficient amount of iron. This nutrient often lacking in the diet of Canadian children; however, it plays an important role in the circulation of oxygen in the blood.

5. How should you discipline a child who plays at mealtimes?

Discipline at mealtimes is no different from discipline in any other of the day's activities. It implies calm and consistent authority on the part of the parents. It does not mean strict regimentation, but rather the acceptance of certain rules.

Mealtimes should be occasions for relaxation and family conversation — but not for playing. The child who has had a rest before his meal will be less excitable at the table, and if the meal is prolonged with a lot of adult conversation, the child should be allowed to leave the table.

6. How can one reduce a child's sugar consumption?

The solution is simple: don't give him any!

The sugar in candies, carbonated beverages, and other sweets supplies calories which provide the child with "temporary" energy, but do not promote growth or keep one fit. An over-consumption of sweets interferes with a child's appetite and promotes tooth decay. Parents themselves are largely responsible for the problem; they confer all kinds of powers on sugar!

"You've been such a good boy, here's a candy."

"Here have a piece of chocolate. It'll make you feel better."

"You don't like your carrots? — Try them with a bit of sugar."

"Isn't plain grapefruit bitter?"

"Here's a bit of sugar, now finish your cereal!"

"Sweetened orange juice is so much better!"

"A meal without a nice sweet dessert just isn't a proper meal."

"My child drinks milk only likes chocolate milk".

These comments illustrate how parents can inculcate a taste for sugar, however unconscious it may be. Sugar has insidiously invaded our eating habits. The consumption of 110 lb. (50 kg) yearly, per person, in North America, is too much!

We must act now to instill new family eating habits, and help our children rather than punish them by eliminating sweets as a "reward and punishment" tactic.

Will a child easily accept this change if he sees his parents eating sweets while watching television at night?

Good resolutions are made together as a family! You should:

- do away with temptation — do not buy any more candies
- gradually decrease sweet desserts and replace them with fruits
- avoid giving sugar an "emotional" value (reward, consolation, pleasure, or a treat).

A young child who learns to savor and appreciate the true taste of fruit, vegetables, and milk will not become a slave to sugar.

Prevention is better than cure!

7. Is it dangerous to drink too much milk?

Some children drink too much milk, and this can have some adverse effects. Milk is very nourishing, but it is not a "perfect" food. As mentioned previously, a vitamin D supplement has to be given as early as three weeks of-age to complete the milk diet. As the child grows, milk is less and less able to supply all the essential nutrients. It is particularly deficient in iron and vitamin C.

A child who drinks too much milk, that is a good deal more than the recommended amount (20 oz. (625 mL) a day) will not be hungry. He will nibble at mealtime and will not eat the right amount of meat, vegetables, fruit, or cereals, and runs the risk of becoming anaemic.

Milk is an important part of a balanced diet. However, it must work with other foods in order to fulfill its role properly. Drinking too much milk is a bad habit which can be corrected as follows:

- by decreasing milk consumption between meals and replacing it with fruit juice or even water
- by offering the glass of milk at the end of the meal rather than at the beginning.

Health Inquiries

1. The child who is allergic to milk.

Many mothers think that their child is allergic to milk, when in fact the problem lies elsewhere. Seventy-five percent of mothers are wrong in their assessement. In fact, only 0.3% to 7% of infants are allergic to milk. A baby who vomits after feeding is not allergic to milk. He has perhaps drunk too rapidly without stopping to burp. Normal feeding time is between 20 and 30 minutes.

The newborn baby who suffers from cramps may "temporarily" exhibit an intolerance to milk, but he is not allergic to it. A mother who changes a baby's formula every few weeks without consulting her doctor is not solving the problem of milk intolerance but rather is interfering with her child's normal digestion.

A baby who is really allergic to milk can still grow normally thanks to various milk-free formulas. Soya-based or meat-based formulas such as HSC Lambs base, Nutramigen, Neo-Mullsoy, Sobee, Prosobee, Similac, and Isomil are a few examples. A family physician or pediatrician is the only one qualified to diagnose a milk allergy and consequently suggest an appropriate formula for the baby.

2. The constipated child.

A proper diet can play an important role in the treatment of chronic constipation.

Certain foods containing cellulose, help normal intestinal functions: bran cereals, whole-grain cereals, raw fruit and vegetables, and dried fruit (prunes, raisins, dates, figs). A child who drinks too much milk and does not consume the proper amount of fruit and vegetables may well become constipated.

Physical exercise and adequate consumption of liquids (water and fruit juice) will also help combat constipation. The use of laxatives is not recommended since they make the intestines "lazy."

3. The child who suffers from diarrhea.

Diarrhea is always a serious problem, more so in an infant than in a preschooler. In all cases, it is better to consult with the family doctor to ensure that proper treatment is received.

A child who consumes too much sugar, or is over-excited, is a likely candidate for diarrhea.

4. The child who has an upset stomach.

It is recommended that a doctor be consulted whenever a small child (from birth to two years) suffers from indigestion.

After this age, the usual treatment is a prolonged fast (½ to 1 day) after vomiting has ended. This gives the tired stomach a rest.

A few sips of mineral or tap water every half-hour will quench the child's thirst. Solids are gradually introduced in the days that follow. Semi-solid foods which are easy digest are first introduced: strained, cooked cereals; toast; soft-boiled egg; custards; ripe banana; apple sauce.

5. The child who is too thin.

As we saw in Chapter Fourteen, the one-and-a-half-year-old to six-year-old child grows erratically. Because of these growth spurts and slowdowns, the preschooler does not maintain a constant level of appetite. His appetite is capricious and he seldom has much reserve of fat especially if the child is very active. When a child suddenly starts to grow rapidly he is unable to put on enough weight to balance the growth spurt in height.

This is no cause for alarm! The situation can be improved by controlling both the child's activity and his nutritional intake. By decreasing his level of activity and increasing the number of calories in his diet, he will be able to gain weight.

Up to the age of six, a child needs a certain amount of sleep to allow him to recuperate both physically and emotionally. If the "thin" child never rests during the day, and goes to bed at the same time as his parents at night, it is obvious that he is overexpending his energy and he is unable to build up his fat reserves!

Without imposing a daily nap on a child, it should be possible to arrange for a period of at least one hour in the day during which he can rest physically and emotionally by listening to a story, coloring, or listening to records. Bedtime can be advanced in order to increase the child's sleep time. It should not be forgotten that a tired child has less appetite than one who is well rested. In addition, the child should probably receive more calories. A review of his eating habits is essential:

• Does the child eat at mealtime?
• Does he eat large or small quantities?
• Does he snack between meals?
• Does he like many different kinds of foods?
• How much does he eat in one day?

A precise answer to each of his questions will enable a parent to develop a plan to enrich a child's diet.

If the child is a small eater, you must bear in mind that regular mealtimes promote a better appetite, and that snacking between meals merely reduces it.

If, on the other hand, he is a big eater, you must enrich his menus in order to increase the number of calories without increasing the quantity of food he eats.

At breakfast, for example:
• cook his cereals with whole milk rather than with water
• serve him omelettes or scrambled eggs instead of soft-boiled or poached eggs
• offer him muffins or brioches instead of plain toasted bread
• give him whole milk instead of 2% milk.

At other meals:
• serve milk-based or cream soups instead of bouillons, consommés, or vegetable juice
• serve meat, poultry, or fish with a white or brown sauce

- serve mashed potatoes (with milk and butter) instead of plain, boiled, or baked potatoes
- dress salads with sour cream or thick dressings
- add butter to the vegetables
- give him bread, biscuits, and desserts made of milk between meals, if he is still hungry
- offer him milkshakes (milk, fruit, and ice cream), etc.
- prepare cookies made with dried fruit and nuts.

A daily walk in fresh air will also stimulate his appetite!

6. The fat child.

Before the age of six, the fat child is less common than a thin one. It is important to remedy this situation before it is too late.

In Canada, 30% of adolescents, 43% of adults between 20 to 39 years of age, and 63% of adults between 40 to 65 years are overweight.

This is a sobering situation especially when one considers that obesity in the adult increases his chances of such illnesses as hypertension, diabetes, and atherosclerosis.

An annual visit to the pediatrican or to the family doctor will enable parents to follow and review their child's weight curve. If he is found to be overweight it will be necessary to try and have him lose a few pounds and change his life-style as well as his eating habits.

In fact, several studies have shown that an overweight child does not eat more than a normal weight one, but he is much less active.

An overweight child must first and foremost exercise more and . . . watch less television!

Establishing the cause of the overweight is as important as the dietetic treatment for it, per se. A child who eats to fulfill a need for affection will respond poorly to restrictions on his diet, whereas a child who eats a lot simply because everyone around him eats a lot, will react better.

A weight-loss diet for a child of this age will hardly be noticed if the mother plans it carefully. Calories are decreased only slightly because the high requirements for growth must be met. A loss of 1 to 2 lb. (½ to 1 kg) per week is sufficient.

The basic foods should never be eliminated: milk, meat, fruit, vegetables, and cereals. On the other hand, lower calorie substitutes may be used, as long as nutritional quality is not sacrified. Useless or superfluous foods, such as candies and potato chips, can always be eliminated.

A child will lose one pound (½ kg) per week be replacing daily:

- instead of 20 oz. (625 mL) whole milk, serve 20 oz. (625 mL) skim milk
- instead of a rich snack (date squares), serve a fruit (1 apple)
- instead of a rich dessert (½ cup or 125 mL) ice cream, serve a fruit (1 peach).

A reduction of 500 calories daily provides a painless way to lose weight.

The mother of a child who is prone to gaining weight should watch very closely the quality and the quantity of the food she serves her child. She must also be aware that the cooking method affects the number of calories in the food served. Fried foods or foods cooked in butter supply more calories than grilled or steamed foods.

Thanks to parental foresight, the overweight child who adopts a healthier life-style (better balanced diet and increased physical activity) before the age of six, is ensuring himself a happier and healthier life!

CHAPTER SIXTEEN

Knowledge Leads to Love

THE FIRST FEW years of a child's life are the years in which he explores the world around him. They are years filled with new visual, auditory, gustatory, and olfactory experiences.

A child slowly discovers colors, textures, shapes, smells, and tastes. After the first few months, his eyes are attracted to the "red" toy rather than the little beige dog, to the orange carrot, rather than green beans. His fingers react to different textures and can differentiate between a plush doggy, a smooth ball, and a rag doll. His taste buds experience a whole range of new tastes and even at this age, he makes his likes and dislikes known (mashed bananas are eaten faster than pureed meats). His ears recognize the music-box's melody. His nose learns to sniff and enjoy pleasant smells.

Everything that is taken in and retained during the first years of life is accomplished through his senses. The more opportunities a child has to see, touch, taste, smell, and hear, the more he gets to know the world around him and the better prepared he is to deal with it.

Senses must be exercised just as muscles must be exercised. The child grows to love the things he knows: the pretty toy he looks at, the cat he strokes, the melon he tastes, the rose he smells, the song he hears!

Food is a part of the child's world. The more opportunities he has to learn about different foods, the greater are the chances that he will like them.

Always keeping the objective of forming good eating

habits in mind, this last chapter suggests activities, games, and experiences for the child which will enable him to discover and appreciate a wide variety of foods while having fun.

Let's visit the market or the farm . . . (two to two-and-a-half or older)

It is a real pleasure for a child to go to the supermarket with his mother. Sitting in a "silver" carriage, he discovers a whole new world of foods.

This experience can be both pleasant for the mother and valuable for the child, even if it only takes place occasionally.

It is better to go shopping for food after having eaten. This spares the mother the wails of a hungry child. In the same vein, buying sweets or cookies to calm the overexcited child must not be done. If it's time for his snack, a child should be given an apple, or a small package of raisins to nibble on.

During this visit, the child learns by watching his mother fill her shopping cart. In his mind, the food that his mother buys is good food: good for the family and good for him! If all he sees is canned goods frozen foods, and prepared dishes, he will not learn very much and will get a very poor idea of what constitutes a good diet.

If, on the other hand, the mother buys basic foods (meat, fruit and vegetables, cereals, and milk products), and she explains why she is buying such-and-such a vegetable or cut of meat (to make a salad, to prepare some casserole), he will feel he is actively participating and this will make him very happy. Every now and then, he should be allowed to make the choice himself between two kinds of cheeses, two vegetables or two fruits, or fruit juice of equal nutritional value. If he has had a say in the actual choice of the food, he will be interested in getting to know it, and will hardly refuse it when it appears on his plate.

The fruit and vegetable market
(suitable for a three-year-old)

A family visit to this market at the height of the season is a treat which should be fully taken advantage of. Between June and mid-October, it is possible to purchase fruits and vegetables in an open-air market. This is one activity a child should not miss.

He can savor the smell of fresh fruits and vegetables, and will learn to recognize the characteristics of good vegetables or fruit: the whiteness of the cauliflower, the firmness of green peppers, the shiny skin of egg-plants and zucchini, the deep colors of strawberries, and so on.

What a pleasure to taste the first carrots of the season!

There is no substitute for the smell of vegetables and fruits in season and this is the perfect way to give our children a taste for them.

The fish market
(suitable for three-year-olds or older)

The fish market presents nature's wonders to the curious and attentive child. No need to visit the ocean to see molluscs or crustaceans, mussels, clams, oysters, scallops, or snails. How surprising to see "green" lobsters swimming in salt water tanks and yet find them "red" in the refrigerated display section. Or how about discovering frog's legs . . . or better still, an octopus!

Fish is no exception to the rule. A child will like it if he has acquired a taste while very young and if his mother prepared it so that all its flavor is retained.

To double this pleasure, let the child choose his own favorite fish once in a while!

The farm (suitable for three-year-olds and over)

To gather a still-warm freshly laid egg in the hen house, to see a cow being milked, to discover a pig's curly tail, to run in wheat fields, to go to a corn roast, to climb an apple tree and pick a ripe apple — these are but a few of the experiences which teach a child about the origins of his food. Throughout the summer, many farms open their doors to welcome families interested in sharing these experiences firsthand.

A walk in the country (for three-year-olds or older).

With a pair of good sharp eyes, and a little luck, one can usually discover several edible plants growing wild during a simple walk in the country. Every month of the summer has something different to offer. In May, you will find the young shoots known as "fiddleheads," a delicious and tender vegetable which is cooked in the same way as green string beans. In June, dandelion greens make an excellent salad and are rich in vitamin C. July brings wild strawberries and wild raspberries. In August, tiny delicious, flavorful blueberries are available. Autumn brings various nuts, walnuts, and hazel nuts which are simply delicious — not to mention chestnuts.

A child soons learns to appreciate the flavor of these edible wild plants which he has picked for himself in the countryside.

Let's try planting our own vegetables

All that is needed to grow one's own vegetables is earth, water, sunshine, and a lot of tender love and care. Even in the heart of the big city, a child can still enjoy the joys of a vegetable garden.

Cherry tomatoes (for three-year-olds and older)

At the end of March, cherry tomato plants are available at horticulturists. They can be planted in a ten-inch (25 cm) diameter pot; the pot is then placed in a sunny window. The aspiring young gardener is then responsible for its care and watering — carefully and tactfully guided and supervised of course. When the warm weather arrives, the pot is put outdoors on a terrace or balcony in a sunny spot. The plants can then be trained to climb on a trellis or stake. If the young gardener has done his job well, he can proudly harvest and eat several miniature tomatoes.

Little peas grow into big peas (for three-year-olds or older)

By sowing green peas, the child is able to observe every step in the development of a vegetable: seed, leaves, flowers, pods, and the green peas themselves. This experience is truly worthwhile!

As soon as spring has arrived, a child can sow two or three small peas seeds in a ten-inch (25 cm) diameter pot, filled with planting soil. Place the pot near a sunny window and water regularly when the soil becomes dry.

At the end of a few weeks, the child will notice the seedling and then some leaves. As soon as it is warm enough outside, place the pot in a warm sunny corner of the garden or outside on the balcony, near a fence or a trellis, since this is a climbing plant.

The child will then be able to watch the successive stages of its growth — the flowers, and then the pods, inside which the peas themselves will slowly form.

Words can hardly express a child's happiness as he tastes the peas (raw or cooked) which he himself planted.

Let's make homemade bread (activity for a four-year-old and older)

What a thrill to discover in your own kitchen that yeast makes dough rise! And what a splendid smell hot bread has as it comes from the oven. What can be more lovely than devouring it warm!

A child who has walked in a wheatfield, has watched the grain being ground, and has helped to make the bread, has had a unique and unforgettable experience!

Bread-making is simple. However, four hours have to be set aside for the dough to rise and for the baking. Early morning or early afternoon is the ideal time to start work on the recipe which follows. The baking will coincide with mealtime so that tasting the bread will not spoil a child's appetite.

Whole-Wheat Bread

Ingredients
5 to 6 cups (1.2 to 1.5 L) whole-wheat flour
1 cup (250 mL) boiling water
2 teaspoons (10 mL) salt
1 tablespoon (10 mL) margarine
5 tablespoons (75 mL) powdered skim milk
¼ cup (60 mL) honey
¾ cup (180 mL) cold water
1 envelope of yeast sprinkled over ¼ cup (60 mL) lukewarm water

Preparation (the mother should carry out the six first steps)
1. Place honey, margarine and salt in a large bowl.
2. Pour in boiling water and mix well.
3. Add cold water and mix until preparation is lukewarm.
4. Add the soaked yeast and three cups (750 mL) flour (1 cup (250 mL) at a time). Mix until mixture is smooth.
5. Add powdered milk and beat for two minutes.
6. Add remaining flour and mix well.
7. Knead dough. Show the child how to do this and let him try if for a few minutes.
8. When the dough has been well kneaded, brush a little vegetable oil over the top of the dough, cover with a damp cloth, and let the dough rise until it has doubled in volume.
9. Once the dough has doubled, show the child the change; let him punch the dough in the center and watch it sink down.
10. Knead dough again with help of the child, shape into two small loaves. Place in well-greased bread tins, cover, and let rise until double in volume. Alternatively: divide the dough into small pieces and let the child "sculpt" his own little loaves. Cover with a damp

cloth and let rise until double in volume in a draughty area, while explaining to the child what yeast is and how it makes the dough rise.

11. When the dough has doubled in bulk, cook in a 350°F (180°C) oven until the loaves are golden and crusty (45 to 60 minutes).

RECIPE INDEX

Vegetable Purees

Fruit Purees

Meat, Poultry, or Fish Purees

Snacks and Drinks

Vegetarian Recipes

GENERAL INDEX

Abrahamson, L. et al. "Protein Quality of Home Prepared and Industrially Produced Baby Foods." *Nutritional Metabolism* 21, suppl. 1, (1977).

Abrahamson, L. "The Mother's Choice of Food for Herself and Her Baby." In *The Mother-Child Dyad Nutritional Aspects, Symposium of the Swedish Nutrition Foundation XIV.* Stockholm: Almquist and Wiksell, 1979.

Addy, H.L.J. "The Breast-Feeding of Twins." *Env. Child Health* no. 21 (1975).

Almroth, S.G. "Water Requirements of Breast-Fed Infants in a Hot Climate." Proceedings Western Hemisphere Nutrition Congress V, AMA 1978.

Anderson, T.A. "Commercial Infant Foods — Content and Composition." *Pediatrics Clinic of North America* 24 (February 1977).

Applebaum, R.M. "Breast-Feeding and Drugs in Human Milk." *Keeping Abreast Journal* 2 (1977).

Applebaum, R.M. "The Obstetrician's Approach to the Breast and Breast-Feeding." *Journal of Reproductive Medicine* 14 (March 1975).

Arnoon, S.S. et al. "Honey and Other Environmental Risk Factors for Infant Botulism." *The Journal of Pediatrics* 94 (February 1979).

"Aspartame and Other Sweeteners." *The Medical Letter* 24 (1982).

Astier-Dumas, M. "Laits pour bébé." *L'Alimentation et la Vie* 64 (1976).

Atkinson, S.A. "Chemical Contamination of Human Milk: A Review of Current Knowledge." *Journal of the Canadian Dietetic Association* 40 (July 1979).

Atkinson, S.A. "Factors Affecting Human Milk Composition." *Journal of the Canadian Dietetic Association* 40 (July 1979).

Atkinson, S.A. et. al. "Effect of Premature Birth on Total and Mineral Concentration in Human Milk." Proceedings Western Hemisphere Nutrition Congress V, AMA 1978.

Barnes, L.A. "Les transitions alimentaires de la première année." *Dialogues en Nutrition Infantile, Health Learning Systems* 1 (1977).

Beaton, G.H. "Nutritional Needs of the Pregnant and Lactating Mother." In *The Mother-Child Dyad-Nutritional Aspects, Symposium of the Swedish Nutrition Foundation XIV.* Stockholm: Almquist and Wiksell, 1979.

Blanchet, M. "Influence des politiques gouvernementals sur la santé maternelle." Congrès de l'Association des Gynécologues Obstétriciens du Quebec, October 1978.

Brault-Dubuc, M. "Nutrition du nourrisson." *Canadian Family Physician* 24 (1978).

Brault-Dubuc, M. "La fer, problème d'absorption, problème de carence." Le *Médécin du Québec* 14 (1979).

Brault-Dubuc, M. "Alimentaire du nourrisson canadien-francaise de la naissance à six mois." *A.C.F.A.S.* 44 (1977).

Brault-Dubuc, M. "Les habitudes alimentaires pendent la première année de vie et les besoins de supplements." *La Lettre: Corporation Professionnalle des Diététistes du Québec* 3 (1978).

"Breast-Feeding: What Is Left Besides the Poetry?" *Pediatrics* 62 (October 1978).

Brown, L.W. "Commentary: Infant Botulism and the Honey Connection." *The Journal of Pediatrics* 94 (February 1979).

Bruch, Hilde. *Eating Disorders.* New York: Basic Book Publishers, 1973.

"Caffeine's Role in Birth Defects." *Nutrition Action:* October 1978.

Calabrese, Edward G. "Polychlorinated Biphenyls." In *Nutrition and Environmental Health, Vol. 1, The Vitamins.* New York: John Wiley and Sons, 1980.

Canadian Pediatric Society Nutrition Committee. "Infant Feeding." *Canadian Journal of Public Health* 70 (1979).

Chandra, R.K. "Immunological Aspects of Human Milk." *Nutrition Reviews* 36 (September 1978).

Chernoff, G.F. "Moderate Drinking May Damage Unborn Babies." Fifth International Conference on Mental Defects, Montreal, 1977.

Committee of Environmental Hazards. "PCBs in Breast Milk." *Pediatrics* 62 (September 1978).

Committee on Nutrition, American Academy of Pediatrics. "Iron Supplementation for Infants." *Pediatrics* 58 (1976).

Committee on Nutrition, American Academy of Pediatrics. "Fluoride Supplements, Revised Dosage Schedule." *Pediatrics* 63 (1979).

Cravioto, J.; Birch, H.G.; Delicardie, E.R.; and Rosales, I. "The Ecology of Infant Weight Gain in a Pre-Industrial Society." *Acta Paediatrica Scandinavia* 56 (1967): 71-84.

Crawford, M.A. et al. "Milk Lipids and Their Variability." *Current Medical Research and Opinion* 4 (1976).

Cunningham, A.S. "Morbidity in Breast-Fed and Artificially Fed Infants, II." *Journal of Pediatrics* 95 (November 1979).

Deeming, S.B. and Weber, C.J. "Trace Minerals in Commercially Prepared Baby Foods." *Journal of the American Dietetic Association* 75 (August 1979).

Delaney, D. *Introduction of Solids in Infancy.* The Montreal Children's Hospital, revised 1977.

Dennis, J.K. "Changes in Body Weight after Delivery." *Journal Obstet. Gynec.* 27 (1971).

"Diet and Iron Absorption in the First Year of Life." *Nutrition Reviews* 37 (June 1979).

Dreikeurs, Rudolf. *Children: The Challenge.* New York: Duell, Sloan and Pearce, 1964.

"Drinking by Mothers-To-Be: A Discussion for Public Health Professionals." *O.N.E. Newsletter,* vol. 1, no. 1 (1979).

Fattah, M. et al. "Breast-Feeding and Its Impact on the Infant's Health and Development." Research paper presented at the XIth International Congress on Nutrition, Rio de Janeiro, September 1978.

Filer, L.V. "Early Nutrition: Its Long-Term Role." *Hospital Practice* (1978).

Fomon, S.F. and Strauss, R.G. "Nutrient Deficiencies in Breast-Fed Infants." *New England Journal of Medicine* 299 (August 1978).

Fomon, S.J. et al. "Recommendations for Feeding Normal Infants." *Pediatrics* 63 (1979).

Foman, S.J. *Infant Nutrition* 2cd Edition: Toronto: W.B. Saunders, 4 1974.

Fomon, S.J. et al. "Skim Milk in Infant Feeding." *Acta. Pediat. Scand.* 66 (1977).

Food and Drug Administration. "Food Additives Permitted in Food on an Interim Basis or in Contact With Food Pending Additional Study." Part 180:37, FDA, Chapter 1, title 21 (1981).

Glueck, S.J. et al. "Plasma and Dietary Cholesterol in Infancy." *Metabolism* 21 (1972): 1121.

Greenwalt, E.; Bales, E.; and Guthrie, D.J. "The Onset of Sleeping through the Night in Infancy." *Pediatrics* 38 (1966).

Greer, F.R. et al. "Water Soluble Vitamin D in Human Milk: a Myth." *Pediatrics* 69 (February 1982).

Groisser, D.S. et al. "Coffee Consumption during Pregnancy: Subsequent Behavioral Abnormalities of the Offspring." *Journal of Nutrition* 112 (April 1982).

Grulee et al. "Breast and Artificial Feeding." *Journal of the American Medical Association* 103:735, 1934.

Hall, B. "Changing Composition of Human Milk and Early Development of an Appetite Control." *Lancet* (April 1975): 779-81.

Hambidge, K.M. et al. "Plasma Zinc Concentrations of Breast-Fed Infants." *Journal of Pediatrics* 94 (April 1979).

Hambraeus, L. "Proprietary Milks versus Human Breast Milk. A Critical Approach from the Nutritional Point of View." *Pediat. Clins. N. Amer.* 24 (1977).

Higginbottom, M.C. et al. "A Syndrome of Methylmalonic Aciduria, Homocystinuria, Megaloblastic Anemia and Neurological Abnormalities in a Vitamin B12 Deficient Breast-Fed Infant of a Strict Vegetarian." *New England Journal of Medicine* 299 (1978).

Higgins, A. "Nutritional Status and Outcome of Pregnancy." *Journal of the Canadian Dietetic Association* 37 (1976).

"Infant Feeding: A Statement by the Canadian Pediatric Society Nutrition Committee." *Canadian Journal of Public Health* 70 (1979).

Jackson, R.L. "Maternal and Infant Nutrition and Health in Later Life." *Nutrition Reviews* 37 (February 1979).

Jakobsson, I. and Lindberg, T. "Cow's Milk as a Cause of Infantile Colic in Breast-Fed Infants." *Lancet* (August 1978).

Jelliffe, B.D. and Jelliffe, E.F.P. *Human Milk in the Modern World.* Toronto: Oxford University Press, 1978.

Johansen, E.; Taves, D.; Olsen, T.O. ed. *Continuing Evaluation of the Use of Fluorides.* Denver: Westview Press, 1979.

Johnson, E.M. and Wchwartz, N.E. "Physicians' Opinions and Counselling Practices in Maternal and Infant Nutrition." *Journal of the American Dietetic Association* 78 (September 1979).

Keeting, J.P. et al. "Infantile Methemoglobinemia." *New England Journal of Medicine* 288 (1973)

Kerr, G.M. et al. "Sodium Concentration of Homemade Baby Foods." *Pediatrics* 62 (September 1978).

King, J. and Charlet, S. "Current Concepts in Nutrition: Pregnant Women and Premature Infants." *Journal of Nutrition Education* 10 (1978).

Klaus, M.H. and Kennel, J.H. *Maternal-Infant Bonding.* St. Louis: C.V. Mosby, 1976.

Klein, R.E. et al. *Symposium on Early Malnutrition and Mental Development.* Stockholm: Almquist and Wiksell, 1974.

Labenthal, E. "Role of the Pancreas in Infant Nutrition and Pancreatic Disease in Children." *Nutrition and the M.D.* 18 (August 1978).

"Lactation and Composition of Milk in Undernourished Women." *Nutrition Reviews* 33 (February 1975).

Lakdawla, D.R. and Widdowson, E.M. "Vitamin D in Human Milk." *Lancet* (January 1977).

Lambert-Lagacé, Louise. *Feeding Your Child.* Montreal: Editions de l'Homme, 1976.

Lambert-Lagacé, Louise. "Le lait maternel, ça coule de source." *Châtelaine* (December 1977).

Lescop, J.L. "L'Allaitment maternel redécouvert." *Le Medecin du Québec* 14 (June 1979).

Letarte, J. et al. "Dietary Effects on Lipid Profiles During the First Few Years of Life." In *Proceedings of the International Symposium on Diet and Atherosclerosis in Pediatrics,* September 1978. Montreal: Carleton Press, 1979.

L'Hirondel et al. "Une cause nouvelle de méthémoglobinémie du nourrisson: la soupe aux carottes." *Annales de Pediatrie* 18 (1971).

Lloyd-Still, J.D. et al. "Protracted Diarrhea in Infancy Treated by Intravenous Alimentation." *American Journal of Diseases of the Child* 125 (March 1973).

Lozoff, B. et al. "The Mother-Newborn Relationship, Limits of Adaptability." *Journal of Pediatrics* 91 (July 1977).

Martinez, G.A. and Nalczienski, J.P. "1980 Update: The Recent Trend in Breast-Feeding." *Pediatrics* 67 (February 1981).

Medina, D. and Nguyen, T.M.N. *Nutrition pendant la grossesse.* Corporation Professionalle des Diètétistes du Quebec, 1978.

Mellies, M.J. et al. "Effects of Varying Maternal Dietary Cholesterol and Phytosterol in Lactating Women and Their Infants." *American Journal of Clinical Nutrition* 31 (August 1978).

Mellon, M. et al. "Effects of Environmental Modification of Atopic Disease and IgE Levels in Infancy." Paper Presented at the American Academy of Allergy Conference, 1976.

Ministry of Health and Welfare, Canada. *Restrictions on the Use of Saccharine in Medicines.* Ottawa, 1977.

Ministry of Health and Welfare, Canada. "Report of the Committee on Diet and Cardiovascular Disease." Ottawa, December, 1976.

Ministry of Social Affairs, Quebec. *Une politique québécoise en matière du nutrition.* Quebec: Document 77-E-425, 1977.

Morse, W. et al. "Mothers' Compliance with Physicians' Recommendations on Infant Feeding." *Journal of the American Dietetic Association.* 75 (August 1979).

Musten, B. "Rickets on the Increase." *Journal of the Canadian Dietitic Association* 43 (October 1982).

Myres, A.W. "A Retrospective Look at Infant Feeding Practices in Canada 1968-1978." *Journal of the Canadian Dietetic Association* 40 (1979).

"NAS Report Confirms FDA Assessment of Carcinogenic Food Additives." *Food Chemical News* (June 1982).

National Academy of Sciences. *Recommended Dietary Allowances, 9th Edition.* Washington, 1980.

National Research Council. *Maternal Nutrition and the Course of Pregnancy.* Committee on Maternal Nutrition, Washington, 1970.

Neill, A.S. *Freedom, Not Licence.* New York: Hart Publishing Co., 1966.

Orga, S.S. and Orga, P.L. "Immunological Aspects of Human Colostrum and Milk, I and II." *Journal of Pediatrics* 92 (April 1978).

Orr, R. and Simons, J.J. "Nutritional Care in Pregnancy: The Patient's View." *Journal of the American Dietetic Association* 75 (1979).

Picciano, M.F. et al. "The Cholesterol Content of Human Milk." *Clinical Pediatrics* 17 (April 1978).

Picciano, M.F. and Guthrie, J. "Copper, Iron, Zinc Contents of Mature Human Milk." *American Journal of Clinical Nutrition* 29 (1976)

Pitkin, R. "What's New in Nutrition?" *Nutrition News* 42 (1979).

Recommended Dietary Intakes for Canadians, Health and Welfare Canada, 1982.

Reeve, L.O. et al. "Vitamin D in Human Milk: Identification of Biologically Active Forms." *American Journal of Clinical Nutrition* 36 (July 1982).

Rowe, J.C. et al. "Nutritional Hypophosphatenic Rickets in Premature Infants Fed Breast Milk." *New England Journal of Medicine* 200 (1979).

Saarinen, U.M. et al. "Iron Absorption in Infants." *Journal of Pediatrics* 91 (1977):36-39.

Saarinen, U.M. et al. "Iron Absorption from Infant Milk Formula and the Optimal Level of Iron Supplementation." *Acta. Pediatr. Scand.* 66 (1977).

Saarinen, U.M. "The Need for Iron Supplementation in Infants on Prolonged Breast-Feeding." *The Journal of Pediatrics* 93 (August 1978).

Sabry, J.H. "Plant Protein in Human Nutrition." *Journal of the Canadian Diabetic Association* 37 (1976).

Sanders, T.B.A. et al. "Studies of Vegan." *The American Journal of Clinical Nutrition* 31 (May 1978).

Satgé, P. et al. "Essai d'un lait 'humanisé' chez l'enfant de petit poids à la naissance — 80 cas." *Annales de Pediatrie* 24 (1977).

Sims, L. "Dietary Status of Lactating Women I and II." *Journal of the American Dietetic Association* 73 (August 1978).

"Special Supplemental Food Program for Women, Infants and Children." Federal Register, *Rules and Regulations*, vol. 45, no. 220 (1980).

Sugiyana, H. et al. "Number of Clostridium Botulism Spores in Honey." *Journal of Food Protection* 41 (1978).

"Survey of Infant Feeding 1975: Attitudes and Practices in U.K. and Wales." Research paper presented at the XIth International Congress on Nutrition, Rio de Janeiro, September 1978.

Thomas, R.M. et al. "Dietary Evaluation of Lactating Women with or Without Vitamin and Mineral Supplementation." *Journal of the American Dietetic Association* 74 (June 1979).

Thomson, C.A. et al. "Current Issues on Infant Feeding." *Journal of the Canadian Dietetic Association* 39 (July 1978).

Tremblay, H. "Bébé: petits pots ou purée maison." *Parents d'Aujourd'hui* 8 (March 1979).

Tremolieres, Jean. *Nutrition.* Montreal: Danod, 1974.

USDA. "Composition of Baby Foods: Raw, Processed, Prepared." *Agricultural Handbook* no. 8 (December 1978).

Villalon, L. and Brault-Dubuc, M. "Evaluation de la diète et habitudes alimentaires de la femme enceinte." *Journal of the Canadian Dietetic Association* 39 (1978).

Vobecky, J.S. et al. "Infant Feeding Practices and Health Status in the First Year of Life." Research paper presented at the XIth International Congress on Nutrition, Rio de Janeiro, September 1978.

Vobecky, J.S. and Vobecky, J. "Nutrition des femmes enceintes; les habitudes alimentaires durant la grossesse et leur changement." *L'Union Médicale du Canada* 104 (1978).

Wei, S.H. et al. "Fluoride Supplements for Infants and Preschool Children." *Journal of Preventive Dentistry* 4 (1977).

Weininger, J. and Briggs, G. "Nutrition Update, 1978." *Journal of Nutrition Education* 10 (1978).

Welch, R.M. and Findley, J.W.A. "Excretion of Drugs in Human Breast Milk." *Drug Metabolism Reviews* 2 (1981).

Whichelow, M.J. "Success and Failure in Breast-Feeding in Relation to Energy Intake." *Proc. Soc.* 38 (1976).

Woodruff, G.W. "The Science of Infant Nutrition and the Art of Infant-Feeding." *Journal of the American Medical Association* 240 (1978).

Yeung, D.L. "Early Feeding Practices, Nutrient Intake and Growth in Infants in Toronto and Montreal." *Heinz Infant Nutrition Update* (September 1979).

Yeung, D.L. "Food and Nutrient Intake of Infants during the First Eighteen Months of Life." In *Nutrition Research* Vol. 2. New York: Pergamon Press Ltd., 1982: pp. 3-12.